Skinny Liver

Skinny Liver

*A Proven Program to Prevent and
Reverse the New Silent Epidemic—
Fatty Liver Disease*

- Eliminate everyday toxins
- Avoid diabetes, heart disease, and excess weight
- Increase energy, vitality, and longevity

Kristin Kirkpatrick, MS, RD

WITH IBRAHIM HANOUNEH, MD

Da Capo
LIFE
LONG

Da Capo Press
Hachette Book Group
1290 Avenue of the Americas, New York, NY 10104
dacapopress.com
@DaCapoPress

Printed in the United States of America

Originally published in hardcover and ebook by Da Capo Press in January 2017

First Trade Paperback Edition: March 2018

Published by Da Capo Press, an imprint of Perseus Books, LLC, a subsidiary of Hachette Book Group, Inc. The Da Capo name and logo is a trademark of the Hachette book group.

The Hachette Speakers Bureau provides a wide range of authors for speaking events. To find out more, go to www.hachettespeakersbureau.com or call (866) 376-6591.

The publisher is not responsible for websites (or their content) that are not owned by the publisher.

Editorial production by Christine Marra, Marrathon Production Services. www.marrathon.net

Print book interior design by Jane Raese
Set in 11.5-point Eidetic Neo

Library of Congress Cataloging-in-Publication Data is available for this book.

ISBNs: 978-0-7382-3464-9 (trade paperback), 978-0-7382-1916-5 (hardcover),
978-0-7382-1917-2 (e-book)

LSC-C

Printing 6, 2021

FOR JAKE & BODEN—

every word I write, every breath I breathe,

and every action I take is for you.

contents

foreword

Michael F. Roizen, MD,
Professor and Chief Wellness Officer, Cleveland Clinic

This book has changed how I think. It's made me realize how important and how easy it is to keep my liver younger so it can keep me younger.

And it has changed how I advise patients. Before 1990, most docs not specializing in liver diseases assumed that the liver was pretty resilient: if stressed by a one-night alcohol excess, it will recover, assuming it's no longer abused with alcohol or hasn't been attacked by a virus. The popular view was that liver diseases only affected people who abused their liver with alcohol or that the diseases were largely preventable. And after all, your liver would regenerate. If you allow me a quick diversion from medicine before 1990 to mythology, I want to quickly tell the story of Prometheus.

Prometheus gave fire to the humans. His punishment from the gods for committing such a crime: the poor fellow was chained to a rock, where a vulture would peck out his liver. Amazingly, his liver would regenerate overnight. We're not sure how the Greeks knew of the liver's power, though it may be because they survived injuries to the organ in battle. While the Greeks were on to something, we're pretty certain that they didn't have as much insight into the liver as the scientific world did in 1990—and does today. The good news is that this myth was largely right. But doctors have also needed to learn a thing or two in the last thirty years.

Up until about 1990 only 1 percent of us suffered loss of energy and vitality due to what we did to our liver with food and other lifestyle and toxin challenges. But that has changed: now 30 percent of Americans are afflicted with fatty liver disease—and with that, a lack of energy and a host of other problems. Remember Morgan Spurlock? In his film *Super Size Me*, he documented a month of eating nothing but fast food. The consequences? His weight and LDL cholesterol zoomed up, he felt lethargic and depressed, and, said one of his doctors, his liver turned into pâté. Now, that might not be the standard definition of nonalcoholic fatty liver disease (NAFLD), but it sure paints a vivid—and accurate—picture of a condition that afflicts a third of all Americans.

In Part 1 of this book, Kristin Kirkpatrick and Ibrahim Hanouneh summarize the full picture of liver diseases and especially fatty liver disease. NAFLD is the infusion of liver cells with fat, caused by insulin resistance, obesity, diabetes, elevated triglycerides, and poor nutrition. As they explain, as you put on weight, your body becomes insulin resistant. When that happens, you can't use insulin efficiently to shuttle sugar into your cells for energy. Instead, sugar gets stored in your liver as fat—and soon you've got NAFLD. And then you are at risk for some major conditions, such as cirrhosis or liver cancer.

Making the lifestyle changes that appear in the plan in Part 2, such as the suggestions for avoiding fast food (remember Morgan!), and learning how to prepare "love your liver" foods inexpensively and quickly will help you become less insulin resistant and thin that fatty liver (and yes, you will learn why eating liver may be one of the worst choices you can make for the health of your liver!). You can continue to make your liver healthier—and lose waist and weight—by following the simple Skinny Liver Plan in Part 3. You'll learn the basics to make and keep your liver skinny—and give you more energy every day.

Kristin Kirkpatrick with Ibrahim Hanouneh have taught me how to treasure my liver, why that is so important, and what to do to keep it young. This is great news for all of us, since what keeps your liver young keeps your brain, heart, eyes, and even sex organs functioning better. This book gives you the plan for a life filled with energy. I'm sharing this plan with my own patients. In the end—if you understand their principles and follow their plan, too—you will be well on your way to making your liver skinny and your life longer and filled with much more energy and fun.

A Healthy Liver Promotes a Healthy Life

*Indifference and neglect often do much more
damage than outright dislike.*
      —J. K. ROWLING

If I asked you to pause for a moment to think about the organs that
are vital to your survival, your heart, lungs, and brain would probably come to mind. That's as it should be, because without these organs, you simply wouldn't be alive. But there's a key player missing
from that essential list: the liver, which is often overlooked in importance, even though it is among the hardest working organs in our
body. Many of us don't have a clue where our liver is, let alone what it
does. In a way, the liver is like the late comedian Rodney Dangerfield,
who frequently complained, "I don't get no respect!" The liver generally doesn't get the respect or attention it deserves until something
goes wrong.

Yet the liver is also like the great and powerful Oz, in that it makes
magic happen from behind the curtain. If you were to picture what
happens in your body as a Hollywood movie, your heart and brain
would be among the lead actors but the liver would be the director.
It's a silent player behind the scenes, but a powerful one that orches-
trates a variety of critical body functions. Located on the right side of
the upper abdomen, just below the diaphragm, the liver is one of the
largest organs in the body (an adult liver weighs about 3 pounds). It
performs more than three hundred tasks, including playing a role in
such crucial metabolic processes as converting the nutrients in our
diet into substances our body can use and store for energy and removing harmful substances from our blood.

While the liver is tough and resilient, the punishment of our modern lifestyle can wreak havoc on this precious organ—and we may not even realize it's happening! Symptoms of liver disease may be subtle to nonexistent until the condition has reached a severe stage, by which point it may be too late to reverse it. Because mild liver dysfunction is often discovered incidentally through elevated liver enzyme levels on a blood test, and because it doesn't cause alarming symptoms the way heart disease does, most of us don't give a second thought to our liver's well-being or give our liver the TLC it deserves. Many people think of liver disease as related to consuming too much alcohol—but that's only part of the story.

The reality is, a silent health crisis is under way, one that affects 30 percent of people in the United States. You may not have heard of it, but you could be among the potential victims. The crisis relates to a condition called nonalcoholic fatty liver disease (NAFLD), which involves an accumulation of fat deposits (particularly triglycerides) in the liver tissue. Largely related to our nationwide obesity epidemic, it's a disease that's alarmingly on the rise; its prevalence has more than doubled since 1988. Yet, because NAFLD doesn't produce symptoms in the early stages, it often goes undetected until it has progressed to nonalcoholic steatohepatitis (NASH), a more serious condition that results in inflammation and, potentially, irreparable liver damage.

In recent decades, we have developed a collective lifestyle that promotes the development of obesity; this has created what's often referred to as an obesogenic environment. This shift in diet and exercise habits, in particular, has given rise to the incidence of these devastating liver diseases. The exponential rise of NAFLD has paralleled the increase in obesity in the United States—and this is not a coincidence. Both surges stem primarily from an unhealthy lifestyle—too many calories consumed from food (and often the wrong foods) and too few calories expended through exercise. The result: Too much fat in our body, too much fat in our liver, and a serious threat to our health and longevity.

It's a dire picture, indeed, and many people are completely unaware of this looming danger.

Who We Are and What We Do

A brief pause so we can introduce ourselves:

Kristin Kirkpatrick: In my work as manager of wellness nutrition services for the Cleveland Clinic Wellness Institute, I oversee the nu-trition programs, which are focused on helping people lose weight and treating and reversing various diseases. Many of the patients who come to see me are overweight and want to lose weight and/or lower their cholesterol or blood sugar levels; often they don't realize there's another hidden threat lurking inside their body. During our meetings, I usually have the lab reports from their blood work: Physicians often refer patients to me because they have elevated liver enzymes (in addition to their cholesterol or blood sugar abnormalities), so that I can put them on the path to weight loss and better health. These elevated liver enzymes suggest the development of NAFLD, which indicates that their lifestyle habits (such as a poor diet and/or sedentary ways), their body weight, or an underlying health condition (such as elevated blood sugar or high blood pressure) could be putting their health in serious jeopardy. Although I never have patients coming to me, saying they need to improve their liver health, that's where we often need to turn our focus.

Ibrahim Hanouneh, MD, a well-regarded expert on liver disorders, and I met at the Cleveland Clinic where he is an associate physician in the department of gastroenterology and hepatology. There, he sees many patients with a variety of liver diseases. Whereas a lot of patients come to me with the goals of eating healthfully and losing weight, some of them who have NAFLD also work in conjunction with a physician like Dr. Hanouneh who can address and serve their medical needs. I asked Dr. Hanouneh to be the medical expert for this book because he's so knowledgeable about these disorders, what's behind their alarming rise, and what needs to be done to reverse this trend. Having the advice and expertise of both a physician and a dietitian often leads to greater success in preventing and treating liver problems—sometimes two heads really are better than one! In the chapters that follow, you will read patient stories from both of our practices, so that you can gain broader insights into these liver disorders, including their causes and consequences—and see how other people have altered their diet and lifestyle habits so they can protect their liver. I've seen success in many of my patients—the road to change is not always easy, but it is always worth it!

While "detox" diets and other plans are very popular these days, this essential organ is at the root of these purification efforts. With so many people unaware of the threats to this organ, which detoxifies the body naturally, we knew that we had to write this book—to raise awareness of this emerging risk to bodies, minds, lives, and longevity and to give you the tools you need to safeguard your liver's health and help it function optimally. Given how important your liver is to your health, well-being, and survival, it's critical to pay attention to these mounting threats right now—before your liver launches a rebellion. You have the power, the wherewithal, and the opportunity to protect your liver, starting now.

How to Use This Book

In Part 1, you'll discover what a healthy liver does and how your lifestyle could be taking a toll on your liver health, as well as the scope of these newly recognized liver problems and the factors that contribute to NAFLD and NASH. You'll also learn about how to take smart precautions to protect yourself from other liver disorders, such as hepatitis, drug-induced liver damage, and alcohol-related liver disease. Part 2 broadly addresses the prescriptive principles for maintaining good liver health (including improving your dietary and exercise habits, managing your weight more effectively, getting enough sleep and getting a grip on stress, and avoiding toxic exposures) and preventing or reversing liver problems through lifestyle modifications. And in Part 3, you'll find an action plan that will allow you to put these healthy liver principles into action with a lifestyle makeover. Think of this as a fresh chance to give your liver and your body a second shot at better health.

Consider this: If a trustworthy agent offered you a free, comprehensive, gimmick- and loophole-free insurance policy that would likely protect your health today, tomorrow, and for the foreseeable future, would you take it? If a friend gave you a no-strings-attached present of a nonstop airplane ticket to a happy, healthy place you've always wanted to visit, would you accept it? It would be foolish not to say "Yes!" to both propositions, right? With this book, we want to give you the gift of good health—a full understanding of the reasons your liver is so important, vital information you (and many other people) aren't aware of, and concrete steps to help you be the healthiest you can be. Along the way, you'll likely lose weight (if you have extra pounds to shed), have more energy, and make major strides in preventing other life-threatening diseases, such as type 2 diabetes, heart disease, and more. It's an opportunity that's yours for the taking!

part one

Say Hello to Your Liver

chapter 1

Your Body's Hard-Working, Multitasking Organ

NOT LONG AGO, Marie, a 45-year-old mother of two, went to her primary care physician for an annual checkup. She reported being in good health and didn't take any medications on a regular basis, but a blood test revealed that her liver enzymes and triglyceride level were elevated and her HDL (the "good") cholesterol level was low. When her health history was examined further, it became clear that Marie had gained 15 pounds in the previous six months and her body mass index (BMI) was now in the obese category (above 30). This wasn't entirely surprising because Marie had been laid off from her consulting job, was feeling slightly depressed, and she had fallen into a habit of eating poorly and being sedentary over the previous months.

After an ultrasound revealed the presence of fatty deposits on her liver, Marie was shocked to learn that she had a liver disease. Her first question was: "Is a fatty liver bad?" (Yes, it is.) Her second question: "Is it reversible?" (Yes, it is.) That was all Marie needed to hear to feel motivated to start a diet and exercise program, which would reduce fat on her liver and improve her liver enzyme levels.

It's ironic: Some people go to great lengths to "detoxify" their body with cleanses, juice fasts, supercharged smoothies, raw food diets, special teas, and other unproven interventions. They swallow various herbs and supplements in an effort to purify their body from the inside out. They try to sweat out toxins in saunas, steam rooms, sweat lodges, and the like. When they do this, they feel that they're being proactive about removing impurities from their body. Well, here's a newsflash: These measures are of dubious benefit because the liver detoxifies the body naturally and automatically, just as a self-cleaning oven does. The key is to keep it in good working order.

The Detox Organ

Despite people's pervasive interest in ridding the body of toxins, many of us generally don't do much for our liver in terms of everyday care. That's a serious mistake, given everything that our liver does for us. On a daily basis, the two lobes of the shiny, smooth, saddle-shaped organ—which are separated by a band of connective tissue that anchors the liver to the abdominal cavity—perform an astonishing array of functions as part of its 24/7 job description. For starters, the liver serves as a highly complex chemical plant, inspection station, garbage disposal, and filtration system, all rolled into one. The liver filters out 1.4 liters of blood per minute. It converts ammonia, a toxic waste product that's formed from processing dietary protein and nitrogen-containing compounds in the body, into urea so it can be excreted by the kidneys. The liver metabolizes drugs and alcohol and gets rid of the by-products that result from the breakdown of these substances. It removes bad bacteria and debris from the blood-stream, and it breaks down worn out or damaged blood cells.

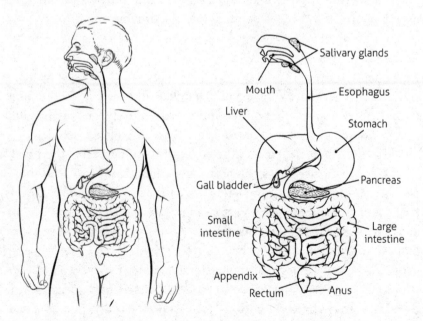

Human digestive system in situ and as detailed view. © Christos Georghiou/Shutterstock

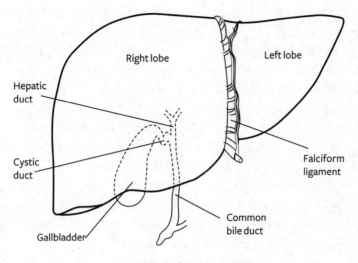

Frontal view of the human liver.

Essentially, your liver—along with your lungs, your gastrointestinal tract, and your kidneys—is detoxifying your body every minute of every day, whether you're awake or you're asleep. No one is immune to the presence of internal (a.k.a. endogenous) toxins, such as metabolic waste products that are generated inside your body, or external (a.k.a. exogenous) toxins, such as pollutants, contaminants, pesticides, food additives, drugs, and alcohol. But having a strong, healthy liver, one that is well cared for and functions the way it should, makes the inherent detoxification process run smoothly and efficiently. If the health of the liver heads south, however, its ability to detoxify your body heads south, too, and no cleanse or juice fast or detox diet can make up for what you've lost with that failing organ.

Your Liver's Role in Metabolism

Moreover, the liver is involved in all of the body's central metabolic processes, including the metabolism of carbohydrates, protein, and fats and the conversion of these macronutrients into forms of energy the body can readily use. When it comes to metabolizing carbohydrates, the liver helps ensure that the level of sugar (or glucose) in your blood stays fairly steady: If your blood sugar level increases (after a meal, for example), the liver removes sugar from the blood and stores it as glycogen (the main source of stored fuel in your body); if your blood sugar level dips too low, the liver breaks down glycogen and releases sugar (glucose) into your blood. As far as dietary protein goes, your liver cells convert amino acids in foods into forms of energy that can be used by the body. And the liver produces bile, a yellowish-greenish-brownish substance that travels to the small intestine where it plays a role in the breakdown and absorption of fats.

Meanwhile, the liver stores fat-soluble vitamins (A, D, E, and K) and vitamin B_{12}, as well as minerals (such as zinc, iron, magnesium, and copper), and releases them into the blood on an as-needed basis. In addition, blood-clotting factors are formed in the liver—these are crucial for preventing excessive bleeding—and the liver helps with the metabolism of sex hormones, including testosterone, estrogen, and progesterone, so that you don't end up with abnormal levels of these hormones. As you can see, the liver is an incredibly hardworking, multitasking organ that never sleeps; it's always on duty.

An Indispensable Team Player

When it comes to organ function, there's often a synergy that's a bit like a well-choreographed dance: if one organ isn't working properly, it can throw the others out of step, too, causing the whole enterprise to function inefficiently. This is true of the liver. For example, the liver works with the kidneys to regulate blood pressure, and it also operates in conjunction with the pancreas and gallbladder to properly digest food; if the liver becomes the weak link in this chain, the whole digestive process suffers. That's just one example of the potential domino effect that liver dysfunction can have.

A few months ago, Robert, a 63-year-old financial planner, had been feeling tired and slightly nauseous, but he chalked it up to stress from work. One night he vomited blood, so he went to the emergency room and was admitted to the intensive care unit. An upper endoscopy revealed that he had actively bleeding varicose veins in his esophagus, a condition that usually occurs in people with liver

The detoxification process that occurs in the liver is far more complex than most people realize, yet it is essential to keeping your entire body functioning smoothly, efficiently, and effectively. At the most basic level, it helps to think of your liver as serving a similar purpose to a high-quality filter in your furnace: By trapping dirt, dust, and toxic particles, the filter allows clean air to be continuously circulated throughout your home, so you can maintain a healthy interior environment. In the case of the liver, here's how this process works:

- In Phase 1, often called the conversion phase, toxins that enter the body are converted into substances that can be excreted through bile (a digestive fluid that's produced by your liver) or urine (which is secreted by your kidneys). Most toxins enter the body as fat-soluble substances, and the liver's job is to transform these substances into water-soluble ones that can be excreted. The problem is, this transformation process can turn these toxins into more unstable compounds that, in turn, form damaging free radicals. Research suggests that proper nutrition—including consuming plenty of antioxidants, B vitamins, vitamins C and E, and carotenoids—is crucial for helping the essential toxin-conversion process in this phase operate effectively and quickly progress to the excretion stage.

- In Phase 2, known as the conjugation phase, toxins are neutralized and prepared for excretion through either urine (courtesy of the kidneys) or bile (thanks to the liver). Phase 2 metabolizes the free radicals that were formed in Phase 1 and prepares them to exit the body. Both phases rely heavily on key enzymes to complete each part of the breakdown process. Research suggests that certain amino acids and phytochemicals (especially plant-based compounds in cruciferous vegetables, such as broccoli, cauliflower, and cabbage) can actually assist with the Phase 2 enzyme activity that converts potentially damaging substances into harmless ones.

- In Phase 3, the elimination stage, the now water-soluble waste products are transported out of the cells and into bile or urine for excretion. This is the clearance phase of the operation, when the body actually says good-bye to those toxins. Mission accomplished!

cirrhosis. Aside from high blood pressure that was well controlled with medication, Robert, a regular exerciser, was lean and quite healthy; a light drinker, he had no prior history of liver disease or a family history of chronic liver disorders.

Yet, an ultrasound of the liver revealed that he had cirrhosis of the liver—which came as a complete shock to Robert—and further tests revealed the culprit: a chronic hepatitis C infection, which was also surprising because he hadn't had a blood transfusion, hadn't engaged in intravenous drug use, and didn't have tattoos; plus, he was married with a monogamous relationship and his wife didn't have hepatitis C. How he was infected with hepatitis C remains a mystery, but Robert apparently had the infection for many years (and had never been screened for it because he didn't have symptoms or clear risk factors), which led to cumulative damage to his liver. Like many healthy people, Robert hadn't given much thought to his liver over the years and he didn't know that baby boomers, born between 1945 and 1965, are now known to be at higher risk of having contracted hepatitis C and should therefore be screened for the viral infection.

As is the case for many people, Robert's first clue that he was suffering from a liver disorder manifested itself in another organ system—the digestive tract. That's because the health of your liver can have a ripple effect on the well-being and functionality of other major organs in your body. Here's a head-to-toe look at how the state of your liver can support or undermine the functionality of other major organs:

Your brain When it comes to normal brain function, the liver may in fact be the most important organ due to its ability to remove toxins from the blood. When this doesn't happen, the brain can suffer the consequences. For example, when the liver is damaged and can't remove or neutralize toxins (such as ammonia) from the blood, the toxins can build up in the bloodstream and travel to the brain where they damage the nervous system. This can lead to hepatic encephalopathy, a loss of brain function; the symptoms can be as simple as mild confusion, mental fogginess, or changes in thinking abilities, or as severe as mental unresponsiveness, slurred speech and movement, loss of consciousness, and possibly even coma.

Your eyes Few people think of the liver when an eye problem occurs, but in some cases, that may be the first place you should look. Several eye conditions can result from the liver's inability to do its job. A condition called scleral icterus, which involves a yellowing of the white part of the eye, can develop if the liver becomes unable to process bilirubin (an orange-yellow pigment that is formed in the liver by the breakdown of hemoglobin and is excreted in bile). Yellowing of the eyes can also be a sign of jaundice, which occurs due to a buildup of bilirubin—and is sometimes one of the first major signs that things are not going well for your liver. Moreover, the liver helps with the metabolism and storage of vitamin A, which is critical for good vision and eye health.

Your thyroid gland This tiny, butterfly-shaped gland in the front of your neck is like command central for the metabolism, growth, and development of the human body, as well as the regulation of critical body functions. Research has found that people who have cirrhosis of the liver have a greater incidence of an enlarged thyroid and that people with hepatitis are more likely to have abnormal results on thyroid function tests. Other thyroid disorders can go hand in hand with chronic liver diseases, as well; for example, hypothyroidism (low thyroid function) is common in people who have autoimmune liver disease (which is why those who have autoimmune liver disease should get their thyroid function checked periodically).

Your heart Because the liver plays a major role in the storage and metabolism of cholesterol and triglycerides (blood fats), it helps keep the veins and arteries that flow into and out of the heart healthy. If it weren't for the liver's ability to break down medications, alcohol, and caffeine, your heart rhythm could become irregular. In addition, research has found that people with nonalcoholic fatty liver disease (NAFLD) are more likely to have heart disease, too, probably due to

THE TRUTH ABOUT METABOLIC SYNDROME

A fancy name for a simple concept, metabolic syndrome is a constellation of risk factors that increase a person's risk of developing heart disease, stroke, and type 2 diabetes. These risk factors include high blood pressure, elevated fasting blood sugar, a low HDL (the "good") cholesterol level, a high triglyceride level, and excessive belly fat (or a large waist circumference). Given the connection to heart disease and stroke, metabolic syndrome is worrisome enough but complicating matters, it also can cause NAFLD—and vice versa. In fact, some medical experts are now calling NAFLD the new face of metabolic syndrome. The two are that closely intertwined!

the fact that a dysfunctional liver increases the risk of metabolic syndrome (see box above).

Your blood Your blood relies on the liver to store fat-soluble vitamin K, which is needed for proper blood clotting; plus, the liver makes key proteins that are necessary for normal blood clotting.

Your kidneys When it comes to removing toxins from the body and preparing them for excretion, the kidney and the liver really do need each other, so it's not surprising that when the liver becomes diseased, the kidney suffers as well. People who have hepatitis C, for example, have an increased risk of developing a chronic kidney condition called glomerulopathy, which affects the parts of the kidneys where waste products are filtered from the blood, thus compromising the kidneys' overall ability to function. Meanwhile, those with chronic liver disease are more likely to have decreased blood flow to and through the kidneys.

Your bones The liver also helps your body absorb important vitamins and minerals—including calcium, phosphorus, and vitamin D—to keep your bones healthy, strong, and happy.

As you can see from this hefty list of responsibilities, the liver plays a vital and indispensable role in your body's ability to function.

Unfortunately, through their lifestyle habits, many people place enormous amounts of pressure on their liver without considering the possibility that this vital organ could get fed up and shut down.

Silent Symptoms, Potentially Devastating Outcomes

More often than not, we are blissfully unaware of the harm we may be doing to our liver until the damage becomes extreme and impossible to ignore. Many different hazards of modern living can take a toll on the health and functioning of your liver. When this indispensable organ can no longer remove waste products, bacteria, or toxins from your blood the way it should, or when its ability to metabolize macro-nutrients and convert them into usable forms of fuel for your body are compromised, your health, energy, and well-being will suffer. It's that simple. And if fatty deposits, inflammation, and scar tissue build up on this vital organ, you can begin to experience severe symptoms, such as persistent fatigue, muscle weakness, nausea, vomiting, ab-dominal pain, memory loss, mental confusion, and other worrisome signs. That's when your liver is sending out serious distress signals.

Among the reasons liver disorders are so often overlooked is that they're often silent in the early stages. Traditionally, liver disease has been linked to alcohol abuse and recreational drug use, which has led to a stigma associated with liver disease. People are often hesitant to see a liver doctor (a hepatologist) or even to believe they might have a liver disease because they're afraid they'll be labeled as a substance abuser. That's certainly not true these days: In the last decade, there has been a dramatic turning of the tide as nonalcoholic fatty liver disease (NAFLD)—which is linked to obesity, diabetes, high blood pressure, and cholesterol abnormalities—has become the leading cause of liver disease in the United States. Yet the public is largely unaware of this connection.

Another blind spot in people's perception of liver disease: There isn't a clear correlation between a person's behavior (aside from drinking to excess) and his or her liver function. By contrast, un-healthy lifestyle habits—such as overeating and getting too little physical activity—can have obvious effects on your waistline and certain aspects of your health. When you consistently eat too much and exercise too little, there's no mystery as to why you can't fit into your favorite jeans. If you start carrying too much weight on your frame, it wouldn't be shocking if you developed joint aches and pains or back problems. If you smoke like a chimney, you know you're at risk for developing a chronic cough. Similarly, most people realize that a lifetime of crummy eating and poor exercise habits, smoking and drinking to excess, can lead to clogged arteries, which can, in turn, cause chest pain, a heart attack, or a stroke (depending on the location of the blockage).

Disruption of normal liver function doesn't typically induce such red-alert symptoms; in fact, you may experience no symptoms at all, which may cause you to conduct your life as though it's business as usual, without giving your liver a second thought. So, while we're all busy thinking about the health and well-being of our brain, our guts, and our heart, the liver is like Cinderella, the poor, neglected step-daughter who does much of the heavy lifting but doesn't get the care or attention she needs and deserves.

The reality is, a neglected or diseased liver can bring catastrophic consequences. The liver is so essential to your overall health that you could survive for only a day or two if it were to stop functioning completely. Instead of exhibiting a smooth texture and a robust color, a diseased liver resembles a misshapen, rotting piece of meat, with bumpy nodules, gristly patches, and scar tissue—it's not a pretty picture! Meanwhile, a fatty liver contains deposits of fat that can cause liver enlargement. If this condition progresses, it can lead to liver fibrosis, where scar tissue forms and further injury occurs to the liver cells. From here, the condition can progress to cirrhosis, which is marked by scar tissue that makes the liver hard and unable to function properly.

Appearances aside, once liver disease crosses a certain threshold, it reaches a point of no return; for severe cirrhosis of the liver, there aren't any treatment options other than having a liver transplant, an extremely complicated prospect for several reasons. It's a situation that adds tremendous angst and anguish to the misery of living with cirrhosis of the liver (whether it's from alcohol abuse, NAFLD, nonalcoholic steatohepatitis, or another disorder), which happens to be the third leading cause of death among adults between the ages of forty-five and sixty-five in the United States. (For more on liver transplants, see box, page 20.) In the meantime, people with chronic liver disease or cirrhosis are likely to suffer from relentless fatigue, weakness, bruising easily, nausea or abdominal pain, abnormal bowel function, difficulty with blood pressure regulation, problems with peripheral muscle strength (which can lead to falls), memory, confusion, and thinking challenges, and other unpleasant symptoms from head to toe. In short, their quality of life takes a serious downturn.

But some liver conditions can't be reversed, including liver cancer, cirrhosis, acute liver failure, and genetic liver disorders, all of which can be remedied only with a complete liver transplant or a partial transplant from a living donor. With a living donor transplant, part of a donor's liver is removed and implanted to replace a patient's diseased liver; after the surgery, the donor's liver regenerates back to its full, natural size, while the new, partial liver that was inserted into the patient grows to a normal size. It's the human equivalent of a lizard's ability to grow back its tail after losing it or having it amputated—nothing short of amazing! Still, it's best to take whatever precautions you can to safeguard the health and integrity of your liver so that you don't have to consider the possibility of going down the transplantation or regeneration path.

The Only Organ That Can Rebuild Itself

The good news is, if they're caught early enough, certain liver diseases—such as NAFLD, alcoholic fatty liver disease (AFLD), and hepatitis A, B, and C—can be reversed with the proper interventions. The liver is the only organ that can regenerate itself: If 25 percent of your liver is healthy and unscarred, the liver can rebuild itself using its own cells and replace the tissue that was lost to disease until the organ returns to its original size. Once cell proliferation is completed, the new cells undergo restructuring with the formation of new blood vessels so as to supply the new cells with sufficient blood flow and nutrients to ensure their vitality.

LIVER TRANSPLANTS

Within the next decade, NAFLD is predicted to become the leading cause of liver transplants in this country, and yet demand will outpace the supply of livers that are available for transplantation. Between 2004 and 2013, the number of adults awaiting a liver transplant due to NASH tripled, and yet patients with NASH are less likely to undergo a liver transplant and less likely to survive for ninety days on the waiting list than are patients with hepatitis C, alcoholic liver disease, or a combination of the latter liver diseases. This is a serious threat, indeed. Many people who have NASH eventually die from complications of portal hypertension, liver failure, and hepatocellular cancer.

Unfortunately, some liver conditions can't be reversed, including liver cancer, cirrhosis, acute liver failure, and genetic liver disorders. For severe cirrhosis of the liver, the only treatment option is a liver transplant, an extremely complicated prospect for several reasons. For one thing, the underlying state of your health will help determine whether you're a good candidate for a transplant so if you have other life-threatening conditions that aren't well controlled, this may not even be a viable option for you. In addition, the cost of a liver transplant, the odds of finding a suitable match (which is based partly on the person's blood type and size), and the recovery from this type of surgery are also tremendous challenges. It also involves a commitment to lifelong medications used post-transplant to prevent organ rejection—and unfortunately these medicines often have severely unpleasant side effects.

There is also an increased risk of kidney problems after liver transplantation. Research suggests that about 27 percent of people who have a liver transplant develop some form of kidney disease and 10 percent of these cases progress to end-stage kidney disease.

Currently, more than sixteen thousand people are on the waiting list for a liver transplant in the United States. They're essentially engaged in a race against time, one that pits the progression of their liver disease against their chances of finding an appropriate match. For more detail on transplants, see Chapter 12, pages 181–189.

The regeneration process can take from a couple of weeks to several years, depending on the extent of the damage. Surprisingly enough, in most cases, liver function is only partially affected during liver regeneration. It's an incredible physiological feat and a critical healing process for people with liver diseases where partial removal of the liver is necessary because of a tumor or chemical injury (from alcohol or drugs, for example). Meanwhile, other liver conditions—such as primary biliary cholangitis, an autoimmune disease that's marked by a slow progressive destruction of the liver's small bile ducts, and hemochromatosis, a condition that causes your body to absorb too much iron from the food you eat—can be managed with various medications and/or lifestyle modifications.

In the chapters that follow, you'll learn more about the latest threats to your liver, the subtle distress signals you should be alert to, and the best ways to protect the health of this vital organ. If you already have a liver disorder, don't despair: You'll also find out how you can set that critical wheel of disease-reversal into motion and improve the state of your current and future health. You will gain the critical tools you need to empower yourself to make liver-boosting changes to your lifestyle, changes that will enable you to better manage your weight, your liver health, your fitness, and reduce your risk of developing life-threatening diseases. These changes will certainly improve the quality of your life—and they may just *save* your life!

chapter 2

The Latest Silent Killers: NAFLD and NASH

C ARLY, 56, came to see me on her physician's advice because she wanted to slim down and get back to her high school weight. During our initial meeting, she mentioned that her doctor had told her that she likely had fat accumulation on her liver because her liver enzymes were slightly elevated; plus, Carly had type 2 diabetes, high cholesterol, and a body mass index (BMI) of 32, which put her in the obese category. When we began discussing the possibility that she might have nonalcoholic fatty liver disease (NAFLD), naturally she was scared, partly because she had never heard of it and partly because she was (rightly) worried that it could cause adverse health events that could threaten her health and longevity.

Many people associate liver problems with excessive alcohol consumption—and that's the end of it; their thinking stops there. Granted, they're not entirely off base, since years of heavy drinking can lead to alcoholic liver disease, including inflammation of the liver and potential scarring (or cirrhosis) of the liver. But there are newer, more prevalent threats to our liver, particularly in the form of NAFLD, a buildup of fat deposits in the liver tissue, and nonalcoholic steatohepatitis (NASH), a more severe condition that involves fat accumulation, inflammation, *and* damage to the liver. These newly emerging liver diseases also stem largely from lifestyle factors, but not usually from excessive drinking; they're more likely to result from being overweight or obese, having poor eating habits, and/or having a genetic predisposition to type 2 diabetes.

For the record, these new threats are in addition to the usual suspects such as hepatitis (A, B, C, and others), alcohol-related liver disease, and primary biliary cholangitis (PBC), a chronic disease in which the medium-size bile ducts in the liver are slowly destroyed, increasing the risk of cirrhosis. They're also over and above the steady occurrence of genetic disorders of the liver, such as hemochromatosis (in which the body absorbs and stores too much iron, which causes liver damage) and Wilson disease (in which the body retains excess copper, which builds up in the liver, causing damage). With most of these disorders, symptoms are typically absent in the early stages, which is part of the reason they go unnoticed for so long.

As Carly's story shows, most people are unaware that having unhealthy eating habits or being overweight can take a toll on their liver; moreover, most people have never even heard of these potentially life-threatening liver diseases. For the most part, research suggests that primary care physicians don't know how to approach nonalcoholic fatty liver disease, either. In fact, many don't even recognize NAFLD for what it is. In a recent study involving 251 patients identified with NAFLD, researchers from Baylor College of Medicine in Houston found that only 22 percent had NAFLD mentioned as a possible diagnosis in their medical charts; all the others simply had notations that their liver enzyme levels were abnormal, they were counseled about making diet and exercise changes, or they were referred to a specialist (such as a hepatologist or a gastroenterologist). The researchers' conclusion: "Most patients in care who may have NAFLD are not being recognized and evaluated for this condition." Compounding the problem is the reality that NAFLD can be asymptomatic even as it begins causing problems for the person who has it.

The Name Game and the Common Denominators

While it's normal for the liver to contain some fat, if fat makes up more than 5 to 10 percent of the weight of your liver, you are considered to have fatty liver disease, which is often noticed by your healthcare professional incidentally when liver enzymes are abnormal on a blood test or fat accumulation on the liver is detected during an abdominal ultrasound or CT scan. NAFLD—which is usually asymptomatic but occasionally causes fatigue or malaise—has become the leading liver disorder in the United States and western Europe, and

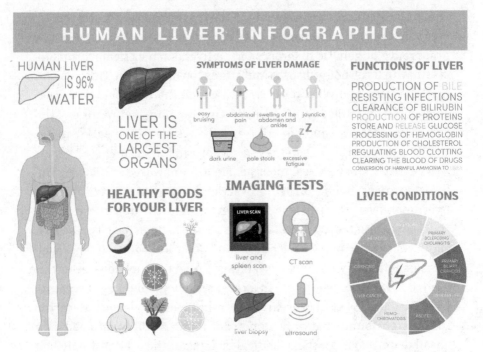

Facts about the human liver. © marina_ua/Shutterstock

in some people it can turn into NASH if it's not reversed. The primary differences between the two conditions is that with NAFLD, there's only fat on the liver; with NASH, by contrast, the liver is riddled with fat *and* inflammation.

As noted earlier, an estimated 30 percent of the US population currently has NAFLD, including more than 6 million children. Meanwhile, approximately 6 million people in the United States are believed to have NASH, and approximately 10 percent of them are thought to have NASH-related cirrhosis. In the last two decades, the prevalence of NAFLD has more than doubled among children, teenagers, and adults, according to several national surveys by health officials. And the rise in NAFLD is parallel and directly proportional to the worldwide increase in obesity, especially abdominal obesity. The fact that obesity rates in the United States and worldwide have skyrocketed in recent decades certainly explains a good proportion of the rise in NAFLD and NASH diagnoses. Since the 1970s, obesity rates have more than doubled among adults and children, according to the National Center for Health Statistics. Among patients with severe obesity who undergo bariatric surgery, the prevalence of NAFLD can be greater than 90 percent.

Some people have questioned whether the rapid rise in the diagnosis of NAFLD stems in part from our increasing awareness of it—the fact that it's now on doctors' radar screens and they're looking for it. And there may be some truth to this because epidemiological studies suggest that NAFLD and NASH are common causes of cases of liver cirrhosis that were described as "cryptogenic" (meaning, "of unknown origin") in the past. A little more than twenty years ago, we learned that excess body fat can cause liver disease and the connections between obesity, diabetes, lipid abnormalities, and fatty liver disease became increasingly apparent.

As you've learned, the liver is a complex organ that wears a lot of different hats, including playing a critical role in the metabolism of dietary fats, carbohydrates, and proteins. In some ways, fats are the trickiest macronutrients for the liver to handle because it needs to metabolize, store, process, and package fat into lipoproteins that can be delivered to cells throughout the body. Although a healthy liver can handle plenty of dietary fat without a problem, the same isn't true of an already distressed liver, which can become overburdened when the person consumes too much dietary fat. If the liver can't handle the overload of fat that's consumed from the diet and accumulated in the body, triglycerides (fats that are carried in the blood) can build up in specific liver cells called hepatocytes, leading to NAFLD. Over time, this unchecked fat accumulation can lead to inflammation and scarring, which progresses from fibrosis (the early stages of scarring) to cirrhosis (the late stages of scarring) of the liver. With cirrhosis, the liver cells are replaced with scar tissue, which impedes this vital organ's ability to work properly.

Other experts contend that the real culprit behind NAFLD is insulin resistance, a condition in which glucose builds up in the blood, increasing insulin levels and triglyceride levels. As you've learned, high blood levels of triglycerides are an independent risk factor for NAFLD because this is the predominant type of fat that builds up in

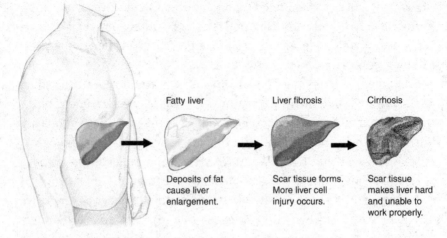

Fatty liver
Deposits of fat
cause liver
enlargement.

Liver fibrosis
Scar tissue forms.
More liver cell
injury occurs.

Cirrhosis
Scar tissue
makes liver hard
and unable to
work properly.

Progression of liver damage from fatty liver to cirrhosis. © National Institute of Diabetes and Digestive and Kidney Diseases, National Institutes of Health

the liver. What's more, elevated insulin levels may inhibit the breakdown of fat in cells throughout the body and stimulate the synthesis of new fatty acids from excess blood sugar. When this happens, the liver ends up with an overabundance of materials for producing fats but nowhere to send them once they're made, so they hang around like truant teenagers and accumulate in the liver, eventually leading to fatty liver disease.

The Next Generation: NAFLD and Children

The presence of NAFLD in children is especially worrisome because their liver is still developing. Recent research suggests that the disease increases the risk of heart disease in kids who are overweight or obese; at this point, no one knows whether NAFLD is simply a marker of an increased risk of heart disease or whether it actually causes heart disease. In addition, unless it's reversed, children will live with NAFLD for longer than adults do, which means there are more years in which it can progress and do irreparable damage.

These days, children are being seen with NAFLD as early as two years old, and with NASH-related cirrhosis as young as age eight. Take a look at what various studies have shown:

- In a 2005 school-based study of obese children in Minnesota, California, Texas, and Louisiana, researchers from the University of California, San Diego, found that 23 percent of 17- to-18-year-olds had fatty liver disease.
- In a 2006 autopsy study, researchers from the University of California, San Diego, examined 742 children between the ages of 2 and 19 who died from unnatural causes; based on their findings, they concluded that approximately 10 percent of all kids in this age group have NAFLD (not surprisingly, the highest incidence of fatty liver was seen in obese kids: 38 percent of them had the condition).
- In a 2009 study of 66 children with nonalcoholic fatty liver disease, researchers from the Mayo Clinic found that NAFLD in children is associated with significantly reduced long-term survival, compared to the expected longevity of the general population of the same age and gender, over a 20-year period; the study found that children with NAFLD have a 13.6-fold higher risk of dying prematurely or requiring a liver transplant.

These are all alarming statistics! In general, NAFLD tends to run in families and often shows up in people who are overweight or obese or have high cholesterol (particularly, high triglycerides); polycystic ovarian syndrome (PCOS), a metabolic and hormonal disorder; type 2 diabetes; or insulin resistance (a.k.a. prediabetes, which is a

THE RISKY BUSINESS OF NAFLD IN PREGNANCY

In a 2016 study involving 1,115 women who had given birth to at least one child, researchers found that those who developed gestational diabetes during pregnancy were two and a half times more likely to develop NAFLD years later. The likely culprit behind the connection: Insulin resistance that developed during pregnancy (the women were free of diabetes before their pregnancies). Because the researchers concluded that gestational diabetes is a risk marker for the development of NAFLD, a diagnosis of gestational diabetes should motivate women to start following a liver-protection plan during and after pregnancy, as well as a weight-loss plan after giving birth. Losing weight during pregnancy is not recommended.

precursor to full-blown diabetes), as it did in Carly's case. Men and those of Hispanic heritage are at particularly high risk. This may be partly because Hispanic people are at least twice as likely as Caucasians are to carry a gene called PNPLA3, which drives the liver to produce excess triglycerides and is linked with an increased risk of developing NAFLD.

Alarming Connections: Piggyback Health Conditions

In many cases, fatty liver disease doesn't occur in a vacuum. Because it often stems from unhealthy lifestyle habits or excess body weight, a number of other health conditions (called comorbidities in medical parlance) often come along for the ride. These include:

Type 2 diabetes The rise of type 2 diabetes has directly correlated with the rise in NAFLD in the United States. The two are perhaps more intertwined than any other disease pair in existence with almost half of all people with type 2 diabetes exhibiting markers for fatty liver; moreover, the vast majority of people with type 2 diabetes are also obese. NAFLD and type 2 diabetes are both closely related to insulin resistance; plus, the liver plays a critical role in the processing, storage, and secretion of glucose. After you eat something that contains carbohydrates, insulin is secreted and glucose is absorbed in the intestinal tract; then it heads over to the liver via the portal vein for the next, and perhaps most important, phase of processing. At this point, the liver stores glucose as glycogen and can administer it to the body when all other energy reserves have been depleted (typically in a fasting state) through a process called glycogenesis.

When too much fat is in the liver, it becomes harder for the liver to do its job and thus it struggles to control fasting glucose levels. The excess glucose causes the pancreas to secrete even more insulin to compensate for the higher levels; this in turn triggers the beginning of insulin resistance and impairment of beta cell function of the pancreas—all of which can lead to the development and/or worsening of type 2 diabetes.

Cardiovascular disease Having a fatty liver is a well-established risk factor for atherosclerosis and premature cardiovascular disease. In fact, the most common cause of death in patients with NAFLD and NASH is cardiovascular disease. Some experts predict that people who develop fatty liver disease are more likely to die of a heart attack before cirrhosis kills them, and the odds grow higher as the fatty liver disease progresses. This elevated prospect of a heart attack begins with the mismanagement of lipids in the liver, which leads to high triglycerides and low HDL (the "good") cholesterol.

In addition, people with NAFLD have been found to be more likely to develop the metabolic syndrome—this relationship is a two-way street, with metabolic syndrome increasing the risk of NAFLD and vice versa. The situation may be even direr for the growing number of children who are developing NAFLD, as some studies suggest that having a fatty liver early in life sets the stage significantly for the development of cardiovascular disease later in life. If this still doesn't scare the bejesus out of you, consider this: People with NAFLD are more likely to die from some form of cardiovascular disease—including atherosclerosis in the carotid arteries, dysfunction of the heart muscle, and vascular problems—than those who don't have NAFLD.

Inflammatory bowel disease (IBD) When you consume something orally, the gastrointestinal system will start working on it; when you absorb something through your skin, the bloodstream may swoop up the substance and carry it along. The commonality between the two processes is that both items—the one that's eaten and digested, and the one that's absorbed through the skin—end up in the liver. I once heard someone refer to the liver as the body's garbage disposal. At first blush, the reference may seem disrespectful, but it actually is fairly accurate. When we put something into our body, either through our mouth or our skin, it has to be metabolized somewhere in order to be used, stored, or excreted.

Several inflammatory bowel diseases (IBD) are associated with liver disease. IBD refers to chronic inflammation of areas within the digestive tract due to the presence of one or more diseases, the most common two being ulcerative colitis (which affects mainly the colon and the rectum) and Crohn's disease (which can affect both the small and large intestines). (Note that IBD is not the same thing as IBS, which is short for irritable bowel syndrome: IBS is a common disorder that affects the large intestine, causing abdominal cramping, gas, bloating, and bouts of diarrhea and/or constipation—but doesn't cause changes in bowel tissue the way IBD does.) Remember: The liver, the intestines, and the biliary system (which includes the gallbladder and pancreas) all need to work together to make the processing of food and the excretion of toxins run smoothly. People with IBD may experience malabsorption and malnutrition issues, which may be another reason why dysfunctions in the gut can often trickle down to problems in the liver. For example, research has found that people with primary sclerosing cholangitis (PSC), a relatively rare condition that involves scarring of the bile ducts that connect the liver and the intestines, are more likely to have IBD; this is especially true in men with ulcerative colitis, according to one study. In another study, when IBD patients were given ultrasounds of the liver, 40 percent of them were found to have fat in the liver. In addition, some medications for IBD may be toxic to the liver. Since the beginning phases of liver diseases can often be silent, meaning they produce no symptoms, people with IBD would be wise to stay on top of their liver function by working closely with their physician.

Celiac disease Celiac disease has been described as a multisystem illness that affects not only the intestines but the organs around it, as well. The connection between celiac disease, an autoimmune disorder, and liver diseases is not well understood—one theory is that intestinal permeability may play a role—but plenty of research has found a correlation. Among people with celiac disease, the most common condition affecting the liver is celiac hepatitis (inflammation of the liver); others include autoimmune hepatitis, PBC, nonspecific hepatitis, PSC, hemochromatosis, and NAFLD.

In some instances, celiac disease has been discovered in people who have frequent abnormal results on liver function tests. Although the incidence of these cases is less than 10 percent, the connection suggests that those with elevated liver enzymes should be tested for celiac disease when other causes have been ruled out. Fortunately, celiac disease can be completely managed with a gluten-free diet, and this treatment frequently returns a person's liver enzymes to normal.

Polycystic ovarian syndrome (PCOS) Polycystic ovarian syndrome (PCOS) affects about 5 million women in the United States. It's associated with cysts on the ovaries, missed or irregular periods, and higher than normal levels of male hormones (androgens). Because PCOS and type 2 diabetes often go hand in hand, PCOS presents an increased risk for fat accumulation within the liver and a heightened risk for further damage with progression to NASH. The reason: Both PCOS and type 2 diabetes are closely related to insulin resistance and central obesity, which increase the risk of fatty liver disease (both NAFLD and NASH). Beyond these obvious connections, the excess androgen levels found in women with PCOS may play a role in fatty liver disease. Given these realities, it's critical that patients with PCOS have regular liver evaluations so they can closely monitor their liver health and the potential progression of a liver condition.

Sleep apnea Studies show that the severity of sleep apnea, a potentially serious sleep disorder in which a person periodically stops breathing for several seconds then starts breathing again throughout the night, may correlate directly to the severity of liver damage in people with NAFLD. As you know by now, there's a strong link between systemic inflammation and liver diseases, especially NAFLD, and one theory is that the lack of oxygen (*apnea* is Greek for "without breath") that occurs when people experience sleep apnea may exacerbate the inflammatory process in the liver. Other studies have found that the lack of oxygen may also increase LDL (the most harmful form of cholesterol) concentrations, another direct link to the development of NAFLD.

Sleep apnea is most common among people who are obese, especially men over the age of forty who also have metabolic syndrome and insulin resistance. Even though sleep apnea is less common in people whose weight is in the normal range, the possible connection between inflammation and insufficient oxygen intake suggests that even people of normal weight may develop fat in the liver and even scarring of the liver if they have sleep apnea. (For more about sleep apnea, see Chapter 5.)

Hypothyroidism Because thyroid hormones are critical to normal liver function, it's no surprise that there's a connection between liver health and thyroid function—more specifically, thyroid *dysfunction*. In particular, hypothyroidism (an underactive thyroid gland) and NAFLD have a clear linkage: Having hypothyroidism may make you more susceptible to a progression from NAFLD to the more serious form of liver inflammation called NASH. Research has found that hypothyroidism is associated with diabetes or obesity and is closely linked to other factors associated with metabolic syndrome, all of which directly ratchet up the risk of developing a fatty liver. Another possible mechanism is that the oxidative stress caused by dysfunction of the liver negatively interferes with the normal function of the rest of the body, including the thyroid gland.

Complex Puzzles of Connected Conditions

A few years ago, Joyce, an upbeat 72-year-old grandmother, had been in good health until family members noticed she'd been getting more forgetful. One day while driving home from the grocery store, Joyce couldn't remember how to get home. She was increasingly forgetting people's names, titles of books and movies, and other things. This was quite alarming to her family because Joyce had always been very sharp, so her daughter and son brought her to see her primary care doctor. Initially, it was thought that Joyce had developed dementia; however, routine blood tests revealed abnormal liver enzyme levels. That's when she was referred to Dr. Hanouneh. An ultrasound of her liver showed liver cirrhosis, which shocked Joyce and her family because she had never been a drinker, had no prior history of recreational drug use, and no family history of liver disease.

What Joyce did have was a BMI of 42, diabetes, and high triglyceride levels—a harmful trifecta that had led to the development of fatty liver disease and cirrhosis. (She had been told many years earlier that she had fatty liver, but she didn't pay much attention because she didn't realize how serious the consequences could be.) Further laboratory tests revealed that Joyce had elevated blood levels of ammonia, a toxin that is normally cleared by the liver in healthy people. In patients with liver cirrhosis, like Joyce, ammonia can build up in the bloodstream and travel to the brain where it can affect memory, concentration, and other cognitive abilities (a condition called hepatic encephalopathy). After being treated with medicine to clear the ammonia from her body, Joyce's mental state improved remarkably.

Complicating the picture, the causation pathway can travel in the other direction, too—namely, with NAFLD increasing the risk of developing conditions that don't seem to have anything to do with the liver. On its own, NAFLD is associated with an increased risk of developing insulin resistance, type 2 diabetes, lipid abnormalities (especially high triglycerides and low HDL cholesterol), hypertension—all of which are hallmarks of metabolic syndrome—and hence heart disease. That's right: You can have NAFLD without these other risk factors and conditions and be vulnerable to developing these other health problems simply because you have NAFLD. It's a tangled web, indeed, and some of these conditions are so intricately intertwined that many people only realize that they coexist, not that metabolic syndrome actually can cause NAFLD or vice versa.

One theory suggests that NAFLD is a "multihit" condition: The first hit comes in the form of fat deposits in the liver, courtesy of insulin resistance. The second hit stems from the liver's response to this stress, namely the release of unstable, damaging molecules called reactive oxygen species (a type of free radicals) and proinflammatory cytokines. A third hit occurs when the oxidative stress that's triggered by these chemicals takes a toll on cell membranes, causing damage. Other potential causes of fat accumulation in the liver include certain medications—such as estrogen (both birth control pills and hormone replacement therapy), corticosteroids (such as prednisone), and calcium channel blockers (such as diltiazem and nifedipine)—as well as viral hepatitis, autoimmune liver diseases, rapid weight loss, and an overgrowth of bacteria in the small intestine (you'll read more about these factors in Chapter 4).

If it's not treated, this cascade of unfortunate events can progress to the liver damage and inflammation that's characteristic of NASH, which in 20 percent of cases can result in cirrhosis of the liver or liver cancer. At this point, the only reliable way to tell if someone has NAFLD or NASH is to perform a liver biopsy. If that biopsy shows that fat is present, the diagnosis is NAFLD; if it shows fatty infiltration of the liver *and* inflammation and some degree of scarring, NASH is diagnosed.

The Progression From NAFLD to NASH

Exactly what causes NASH to develop from NAFLD in some people but not in others isn't entirely understood. According to the American College of Gastroenterology, there are several leading theories, including increased oxidative stress (specifically, the person's body may have an imbalance between the production of free radicals and the ability to counteract or neutralize their harmful effects with antioxidants); the person's inflammatory cells, liver cells, or fat cells produce and release inflammatory proteins called cytokines; normal cells in the liver undergo increased apoptosis (cellular suicide); white blood cells infiltrate fat tissue, leading to inflammation; and alterations in gut microbiota (intestinal bacteria) play a role in liver inflammation.

Whatever the underlying mechanisms are, the result is similar: A serious threat to your health, your well-being, and your life. If NAFLD isn't reversed or managed properly with lifestyle interventions, and if the liver inflammation that occurs with NASH progresses, the consequences can be grim, with the only remaining treatment being a liver transplant. But NAFLD doesn't have to be a runaway train; it can be stopped, and even reversed, with the right interventions.

Reversing the Tide

For these reasons, it's important to catch NAFLD as early as possible and take steps to improve it—ideally, before various lifestyle-related factors can have a harmful cumulative effect on your liver. For example, if you have NAFLD, the following behaviors can increase your susceptibility to liver damage even more:

- Drinking excessive amounts of alcohol on an ongoing basis
- Binge drinking, which is defined as consuming 4 or more drinks for women, 5 or more for men, in about 2 hours
- Routinely popping pain relievers, such as acetaminophen—if you're overweight and have aching joints or chronic back pain, for example

Many experts believe that the first and most effective step in preventing and treating NAFLD is to attain and maintain a healthy weight, which will help you avoid insulin resistance and metabolic syndrome. The best ways to do this, of course, are to improve the quality of your diet (cutting your calorie intake, if need be) and increase your level of physical activity. Besides helping you lose weight, many studies suggest that such lifestyle modifications can have a directly positive effect on the liver by reducing elevated liver enzymes and improving fatty liver disease. Best of all, there's some flexibility in how you can get to that prize: A 2003 review of fifteen clinical studies spanning 1967 through 2000 found that when it comes to NAFLD, a broad spectrum of diets with different calorie restriction intensities and macronutrient composition—including low-carb and high-carb plans and both low-fat and higher-fat regimens—led to reductions in liver enzymes and fat deposits in the liver. So, the good news is that it doesn't necessarily matter what lifestyle or diet plan you choose; regardless of how you do it, upgrading your eating habits can lower your risk.

Research also suggests that when obese people with NAFLD lose more than 7 percent of their body weight, they experience significant improvements in the presence of fat and inflammation in their liver. Because the role of obesity in NAFLD is so intense and powerful, some experts believe that the sooner excess body weight is shed, the better it is for the person's liver. One cautionary note, though: the weight loss should be at a healthy, reasonable rate, as rapid weight loss actually may *increase* the risk of fatty liver disease, as you'll learn in the next chapter. Ultimately, the better-late-than-never principle applies here: it's better to lose excess weight whenever you can than not to do it at all. In some cases, even people with NASH can improve the structure and composition of their liver with dietary modifications, lots of physical activity (on the order of 200 minutes of moderate exercise per week), and other behavior changes.

Remember Carly, the patient who wanted to get back to her high school dress size? After learning that she has NAFLD, she was very motivated to do whatever she could to get rid of the condition. So, I prescribed a diet that consisted primarily of fruits, vegetables, lean sources of protein, and healthy fats, along with a program of regular exercise and stress management. By sticking with the dietary changes, including portion-controlled meals, and walking briskly for forty-five minutes at a stretch at least four times a week, Carly lost 17 pounds over five months, which dropped her from the obese category to the overweight range. The exercise and weight loss also improved her cholesterol readings and boosted her energy. Recently, her liver enzymes were reassessed and they are back to the normal range. Now she is determined to keep them there!

In the coming chapters, you'll discover exactly how you can protect your liver from NAFLD and NASH or potentially reverse these conditions if you have them—by modifying your lifestyle habits. This involves consuming a diet your liver will love—one that's full of antioxidant-rich fruits and vegetables, fish and other foods that are loaded with omega-3 fatty acids, healthy bacteria called probiotics, healthy fats from nuts, seeds, and other sources; limiting your alcohol intake; exercising regularly; and attaining and maintaining a healthy weight. It's also important to get plenty of sleep on a regular basis, control your level of stress (or your response to it), avoid medications that can be harmful to your liver, and steer clear of potential environmental toxins.

This may sound like a tall order to fill, but consider this: Taking these steps will have a positive ripple effect on your overall health, not only because a healthy liver can enhance the functionality of your other organs, but also because the same lifestyle measures that can protect your liver are also beneficial for your heart, lungs, immune system, brain, and other organ systems. (In some cases, medications and/or surgery may be warranted, too, for NAFLD and NASH, as you'll see in Chapter 12.) The point is, if you show your liver the love it needs and deserves, you'll shield yourself from the latest silent killers and the rest of your body will thrive, too. This is an instance where every part of your body wins!

chapter 3

Eat, Drink, and Be Healthier

A YEAR AGO, Terri, 55, came to me, seeking a general plan for weight loss. She had a body mass index (BMI) of 33 and had tried, as she put it, "every diet known to man" without success. Terri had also been diagnosed with fatty liver disease a few years earlier, but when I asked her about it, she said she had never really given it much thought. In fact, since the diagnosis, she had gained about 15 pounds and had stopped exercising. In addition, Terri had a family history of liver disease on both her mother's side (liver cancer) and her father's side (nonalcoholic fatty liver disease, NAFLD). She was particularly worried about following in her mother's footsteps and developing liver cancer, because she wasn't aware that having NAFLD, which related to her excess body weight, could threaten her long-term health as well.

At first blush, the link between obesity and liver diseases may not seem obvious. After all, what does body fat have to do with the liver? Plenty, it turns out. For one thing, when people regularly consume more calories than they expend, that extra energy is stored as body fat in a number of places, including in adipose (a.k.a. fat) tissue, but also in internal organs, such as the liver. For the benefit of their appearance, many people don't want to have a fatty or flabby waistline, but *everyone* should be concerned about avoiding a fatty liver for the sake of his or her health!

In recent years, researchers have begun to tease out the specific lifestyle patterns that put people at risk for these hidden liver disorders. High on the list of offenders: consuming lots of sugary foods and refined carbs, drinking regular or diet soda, and snacking on high-fat fare. In a 2014 study, researchers from the Netherlands found that people who snack in general and snack in particular on high-fat and high-sugar foods have more belly fat and fat in their liver than those who don't munch on this stuff.

People with NAFLD also tend to drink a lot more soda, which often contains fructose, than do those who don't have the condition. A 2015 study from Tufts University found that daily consumption of soda, juice, lemonade and noncarbonated fruit drinks is associated with accumulation of fat in the liver. And a 2010 study from Duke University found that increased fructose consumption in the diet led to an increase in the severity of liver fibrosis (scarring) in patients with existing NAFLD.

Sugar: Alcohol without the Buzz—But with All the Damage

Why does the liver take such a beating from sugar, compared to other essential organs? It probably has everything to do with the fact that the liver is the only organ that can actually process fructose, the sugar found in most sugary and processed foods. It's fructose that's the primary problem, as far as the liver is concerned, and, in fact, changes in our dietary habits over the last thirty years, including substantial increases in our fructose consumption, have paralleled the rise in NAFLD as well as obesity. *A coincidence?* It's highly unlikely!

To put this potential for harm in perspective, here's a quick primer on sugars, how they fit into the category of carbohydrates, and how they affect the body: Carbohydrates are either complex (found in nutrient-dense foods, such as legumes, vegetables, or whole grains) or simple (such as those in processed sugary or starchy snacks, white refined grains, and candy). Complex carbohydrates, which have three or more sugar molecules linked together in a chain, are more difficult to digest than their simpler counterparts, which contain only one to two sugar molecules. As far as simple sugars go, the only redeeming stars nutritionally speaking are galactose in milk and fructose that's naturally in fruit. Fructose and glucose (which is found in starchy carbs) are both simple carbohydrates that are rapidly utilized for energy and trigger quick elevations in blood sugar and insulin levels. As far as your liver is concerned, fructose that's naturally in its original form (that is, in whole fruit) is not a problem, but fructose that's been extracted from fruit and added to processed foods is. Your digestive system can't metabolize the processed forms of fructose well, so while only 20 percent of the glucose you consume makes its way into the liver, 100 percent of your fructose intake does.

While small amounts of added fructose aren't likely to have a huge impact on the liver, excess fructose consumption can overwhelm the mitochondrial capacity in the liver cells; instead of being converted to glucose that your body can use as energy later, that excess fructose is converted into fatty acids and stored as droplets of a particular form of fat, called triglycerides, in the liver. Neuroendocrinologist Robert Lustig, MD, a professor at the UCSF School of Medicine and author of *Fat Chance: Beating the Odds Against Sugar, Processed Food, Obesity, and Disease*, once referred to fructose as "alcohol without the buzz." That's an accurate moniker in terms of the damage it imposes on our liver, because ethanol, the alcohol contained in wine, beer, and spirits, has similarities to the metabolic pathways that fructose takes.

If you overwhelm the liver with too much fructose too often, that overload will create even more fat that will then build up in that organ. Over time, these excess fats will continue to collect, causing liver cells to swell and eventually die. Besides spelling big trouble for the liver—upping the risk of NAFLD, nonalcoholic steatohepatitis (NASH), cirrhosis, and liver cancer—these excess triglycerides also make their way to other areas of the body, including the arteries that lead to the heart and brain, and they set the stage for the development of insulin resistance. Given these effects, it's not surprising that research from South Korea found that people with fatty liver are five times more likely to develop type 2 diabetes than are those who don't have fat accumulations on this vital organ. It's a common finding: In a 2009 study, researchers from Brazil sent 180 patients with type 2 diabetes for abdominal ultrasound scans to look for NAFLD and it turned out that 69 percent of them had it! Besides the direct harm that excess fructose can cause to the liver, a high fructose intake can lead to detrimental metabolic effects that can increase the risk of developing NAFLD—namely, boosting the body's fat mass and systemic inflammation and inducing insulin resistance, which can result in liver damage.

Sneaky Culprits: Saturated Fat and Cholesterol

It's not just your fructose intake that matters; research also suggests that people with a fatty liver tend to eat more meat and other foods that are high in saturated fat and cholesterol. A 2013 review of various high-fat diets found an association with increases in liver enzymes, inflammation, and scarring in addition to other metabolic changes, such as increases in cholesterol levels and body weight. If you were to look at a liver that's been walloped by too much fat and sugar and one from a heavy drinker, they would be nearly indistinguishable from each other.

The 2004 documentary film *Super Size Me* presented an extreme example of this damage in progress: When director Morgan Spurlock spends a month eating all his meals at McDonald's and avoiding exercise, he gains 24 pounds, ratchets up his cholesterol by 65 points, and damages his liver. He later revealed that his doctors said his liver had become "like pâté" because it was so filled with fat. His experience wasn't a fluke. In a 2008 study, researchers from Sweden asked healthy young adults to dine on two fast-food meals per day and shirk their workouts for four weeks. By the study's end, their blood levels of the liver enzyme alanine aminotransferase (ALT) had shot up dramatically. (This is significant because with any degree of liver injury, the ALT enzyme leaks outside the liver cells into the blood, which is why elevated ALT levels in the blood indicate liver damage.)

The obvious offender in these instances is the high fat content in fast foods, but too much protein could be a contributing factor, as well. The reason: When you consume any form of protein, your body produces ammonia, which is a toxin that your liver renders harmless through its natural detoxification process; eat too much protein, and your liver can't keep up with the demanding detoxifying process, which can allow ammonia and other toxic substances to gradually build up in your blood. Over time, an accumulation of ammonia in the bloodstream can lead to memory loss, forgetfulness, confusion, and altered behavior—signs of what's called hepatic encephalopathy. Finally, in addition, a high salt intake (which tends to go along with consumption of fast food) can worsen fluid buildup and swelling in the liver in more advanced cases of liver disease.

Who's At Risk?

Many people don't have a clue whether they are at risk for developing a liver disorder—or whether problems with this overworked organ run in their families. Excessive alcohol intake is the most widely known cause of liver problems—and it is indeed one of the leading causes—but there are many other culprits that contribute to the more than one hundred known forms of liver disease. Generally, risk factors for liver diseases fall into two categories: those you can modify and those you can't. Let's start with the latter because it's a shorter list.

What You Can't Change
Nonmodifiable risk factors include advancing age, gender, a genetic predisposition, and certain ethnicities.

Age Adults over the age of 60 are more susceptible to liver disease, primarily because the efficiency of liver function declines with age, which means the liver has to work harder to rid the body of toxins and other harmful substances. This makes older adults more vulnerable to the effects of liver-damaging toxins (such as PCBs in farmed fish), medications (such as chronic use of acetaminophen), or herbs (such as kava, a nonpharmaceutical approach to treating anxiety). You'll learn more about the damaging effects of these factors in the next chapter.

Gender Because a woman's liver breaks down environmental toxins, some medications, and herbs more slowly than a man's does, women are more vulnerable to certain liver problems. Alcohol is the most well-known example of this, but a similar effect occurs with ingestion of medications, herbs, and some environmental toxins. Female hormones may play a role, as well. Some studies suggest that the amount of circulating hormones, specifically estrogen, at various times of the menstrual cycle may affect the rate at which alcohol or medications are metabolized.

Genetic factors Several forms of liver disease—such as Wilson disease, which leads to a toxic buildup of copper in the liver, and hemochromatosis, which causes excess iron to be stored—stem from inherited gene abnormalities. When Bart, 45, a healthy man with a family and a busy work life, came in for an annual physical, he had no physical complaints aside from mild fatigue, and after the exam, he was given a clean bill of health. But routine blood work found that his liver enzymes were slightly high. The reason was initially a mystery because his weight was in the healthy range, he was a light drinker (who consumed at most a couple of glasses of wine on the weekends), and he had no history of illicit drug use, tattoos (if the equipment used is contaminated, hepatitis B or C can be transmitted in the tattooing process), or heavy chemical exposure. But he did have a strong family history of liver disease: His dad had died of cirrhosis of the liver; his uncle, of liver cancer. Additional blood tests revealed that Bart had elevated iron levels, which raised the suspicion of hemochromatosis, a genetic disorder that causes excess iron to be absorbed and stored in various body tissues, especially the liver, heart, and pancreas.

Excess iron in the blood may not seem like a big deal, but in men in particular it can be serious. Iron in the body is usually toxic, but the body has the ability to get rid of the excess iron and keep only what it needs. It does this through the use of a hormone called hepcidin, which is exclusively synthesized in the liver. While treatable, hemochromatosis can often go unnoticed for as long as a decade, and if iron levels build up and are left untreated, this condition can lead to severe liver damage including cirrhosis, liver cancer, or even liver failure. What's more, having iron overload disease can put you at higher risk for other life-threatening conditions, such as a *Vibrio vulnificus* bacterial infection, which is fatal 50 percent of the time in high-risk people, according to new research from UCLA.

Then there are liver diseases that are caused by the immune system attacking the liver—as is the case with autoimmune hepatitis and primary biliary cholangitis—and some people are simply born with a genetic susceptibility to these diseases. A 2015 study from Japan found that carriers of mutations in the PNPLA3 gene are more likely to develop NAFLD even if their weight falls into the category of a normal BMI.

Ethnicity Those who are of Hispanic descent tend to have a higher risk of developing NAFLD and more severe forms of the disease (Caucasians are second in line). The exact reason isn't known, but one theory is that it's because the Hispanic population has a higher incidence of insulin resistance, high triglycerides, and obesity—all of which are risk factors for NAFLD—than other ethnic groups do. Another theory is that it may have to do with a genetic susceptibility to develop abdominal obesity, which often includes fatty deposits on the liver.

Risks You Can Change

High on the list of modifiable risk factors are obesity and alcohol intake, which are implicated in both nonalcoholic fatty liver disease and alcoholic liver disease, respectively. But there are others, too. Let's start with the big ones (so to speak):

Being overweight While regular physical activity and dietary factors play a significant role in the health and well-being of your liver (you'll learn more about these factors in Chapters 6 and 7), when it comes to the risk of developing NAFLD, your body weight trumps all other influences. However, the tipping point where excess weight becomes problematic may be different from one person to another, depending on genetic influences and other risk factors. For example, someone who has a BMI of 28 (which puts him or her in the overweight category) and a strong family history of liver problems might be at as high a risk for developing NAFLD as someone else who has a BMI of 31 (the obese category), but doesn't have a genetic susceptibility to liver problems.

Excess body weight is a major risk factor for both NAFLD and type 2 diabetes, and it probably links the two diseases through the

THE SKINNY ON BODY FAT

Research suggests that people who are "skinny fat"—meaning, they appear thin on the outside but have substantial amounts of internal fat—are also at increased risk for developing NAFLD. This is especially true if they have a lot of visceral fat that's stored in and around the organs in the abdomen. Unlike the pinch-an-inch type of fat that's stored just beneath the skin's surface (what's called subcutaneous fat), visceral fat can disrupt normal hormonal communication between organs, leading to chronic levels of low-grade inflammation and insulin resistance. In fact, despite having a BMI in the normal range (below 25), people who are "skinny fat" often have the hallmarks of metabolic obesity, such as excess belly fat, elevated fasting blood sugar levels, high triglyceride and low HDL (the "good") cholesterol levels, and high blood pressure. Remember: High levels of triglycerides and low levels of HDL cholesterol are very common in people who have NAFLD.

Even if their weight is normal, people who have these metabolic risk factors should reduce their consumption of fructose and glucose to prevent fat accumulation on their liver. A 2013 study from Wake Forest University found that when normal-weight animals were fed a high-fructose diet, they experienced liver damage even though they didn't gain weight or consume an excessive amount of calories. The take-home message: Keep your intake of added and processed fructose low (remember: the fructose that naturally occurs in fruit isn't a problem) and if your weight is normal but you have elevated liver enzymes on a blood test, you need to look further into the possibility that your liver is riddled with fat. This is especially true if you have excess visceral (abdominal) fat, elevated triglycerides, and low HDL cholesterol.

pathway of insulin resistance. After all, visceral fat (a.k.a. abdominal fat), liver fat, and skeletal fat accumulations each play distinct but overlapping roles in the development of insulin resistance. As previously described, the development of NAFLD is a multihit process and insulin imbalances play a central role in the first insult, setting the stage for factors that promote fat accumulation in the liver to swing into action. This first hit makes the liver cells susceptible to secondary insults from oxidative stress, mitochondrial dysfunction, apoptosis (cellular suicide), and other injuries that can contribute to the progression from fat accumulation in the liver to inflammation and scarring of this precious organ.

As a large risk factor for NAFLD, excess body weight, like alcohol, doesn't take too much above the normal range for damage to the liver to begin. Although the vast majority of people with NAFLD have a BMI over 30 (which is considered obese), the distribution of body fat may be even more detrimental than the number on the scale. People who are carrying extra pounds are often classified as either apple-shaped (with fat in the abdomen, which means close to your liver) or pear-shaped (where fat is distributed in the hips and thighs). If you're overweight, you probably know which type you are. The fat in an apple-shaped body is more metabolically active and it can release fatty acids into the bloodstream, which directly impacts the liver. If your BMI puts you in the overweight category (25 or over) and you carry that excess weight in the midsection, you're more likely to develop NAFLD and subsequent liver damage unless you take steps to control your weight.

Yet, because it's hard to predict who will develop NAFLD and who won't and because obesity's role in NAFLD is so profound, some experts believe that the sooner someone who is overweight or obese sheds excess pounds, the healthier his or her liver will become. (Slimming down if you're overweight will also confer other health benefits to your heart, lungs, musculoskeletal system, and more.) For many people, losing 3 to 5 percent of their body weight is sufficient to reverse or improve NAFLD, but some people with NASH may require a loss of 10 percent to eliminate liver inflammation.

Consuming too much alcohol It's widely known that too much alcohol takes a toll on the liver, but most people don't know why. It's because a steady habit of beer, wine, or cocktails strains the liver, forcing it to work overtime to convert the ethanol in alcohol into less harmful substances that can be removed from the body in urine. Meanwhile, the absorption of alcohol can cause fat to accumulate on the liver and lead to inflammation there. If the damage continues over time, this can result in scarring (cirrhosis) and liver failure.

Many of my patients have asked me how much is too much when it comes to alcohol consumption and their liver. My answer: It depends on your health and what you define as "a drink." Many patients who see me admit that they simply pour until they think they have what they deem to be a "portion," but studies show that eyeballing your drink servings may lead to an underestimation of how much you're actually consuming. The official definition of a serving of alcohol is a 5-ounce glass of wine, a 12-ounce beer, or 1.5 ounces of spirits. Other factors that affect the how-much-is-too-much equation: Are you overweight? Do you have a family history of liver diseases? Does alcoholism run in your family?

Several studies have shown that modest alcohol consumption (less than 20 grams per day), especially red wine, could actually *help* people with existing NAFLD by increasing their sensitivity to insulin and reducing other cardiac risk factors (such as low HDL and clot-promoting elements). Meanwhile, moderate consumption of red wine (up to one glass per day) actually may cut the risk of developing NAFLD by 50 percent, according to a 2008 study from the University of California, San Diego; in this particular study, the results were only seen with wine, not beer or spirits. The perks from red wine may stem partly from its polyphenols, phytochemicals (plant-based compounds) that act as antioxidants and protect liver cells from oxidation and free radical damage. Research indicates that red wine has five times more phenolic compounds than white wine. A 2009 animal study from Portugal suggests that the polyphenolic compounds in red wine may also help offset the damaging effects that alcohol has on the liver.

But other beneficial compounds in *vino rosso* may also play a role: A 2015 study from Oregon State University showed that ellagic acid, a phytochemical in dark red grapes, slowed the growth of existing fat cells in the liver and slowed the formation of new fat cells; it also boosted the metabolism of fatty acids in liver cells in a laboratory setting. Meanwhile, a 2013 study by the same Oregon State researchers found that when overweight mice were fed extract from the grapes that are used to make pinot noir, they had less fat in their liver and better control of their blood sugar level compared to overweight mice that did not receive the extract; both groups of mice were on a high-fat diet. Their findings showed that the grape extracts increased specific protein activity in the liver that helped with the metabolism of fat and sugar—the same mechanism in medications that are used for lowering blood sugar and triglyceride levels. This is a stellar example of how the right foods and beverages can be good medicine!

Yet there is always a flip side in the world of research. A study from 2000 in northern Italy suggests that for obese people who have fat on their liver, having any alcohol at all may be contraindicated (the study found that obese people who drank alcohol had a greater risk of hepatic steatosis, fatty deposits on the liver, than did obese people who did not drink). What's more, a 2009 study from Portugal found that liver disease is the most common cause of alcohol-related deaths, which means that your liver is more likely to kill you if you abuse alcohol than are the odds that a car accident or cancer will. That's a sobering fact, indeed!

It's important to consider gender when it comes to alcohol, too. Simply put, if a man and a woman are each having a 5-ounce glass of wine, the woman will feel it before the man does. So will her body. From a physiological perspective, the woman will actually absorb more alcohol: Because a woman's body contains less water than a man's does, women are not able to dilute alcohol as much as men can, which results in women having a higher concentration of alcohol in the blood. Women may also take longer to rid the body of alcohol, due to smaller quantities of an enzyme called alcohol dehydrogenase, which is needed to break down alcohol. Want proof? Research from the University of Notre Dame showed that a 140-pound man who had two drinks in one hour had a blood alcohol level of 0.38 while the blood alcohol level of a woman of the same weight had one of 0.48. More absorption plus a longer time for excretion multiplied by years of moderate to heavy drinking equals a greater risk to the liver for women than for their male counterparts.

How much and how often you drink can affect your risk of developing a number of liver conditions. Research from the World Health Organization's report on the status of alcohol and health found that daily heavy drinking was the single biggest predictor of developing alcoholic cirrhosis. For the record, the Centers for Disease Control now defines heavy drinking as having fifteen or more drinks per week for men and eight or more per week for women. That equates to just a little over the recommended daily limit recommended by the American Heart Association (two drinks per day for men, one per day for women).

Despite the evidence, patients routinely underestimate their alcohol consumption or justify that drinking alcohol every day is necessary to reap the health benefits some studies have shown. In those who are vulnerable, regular overindulgences—such as having an extra pour at a dinner party or a boozy night out with friends—may be all it takes to catapult a marginally healthy liver to a diseased state. Your best bet is to stick with the guidelines for your gender and limit the number of days each week that you drink alcohol. Measuring the amount of alcohol in the glass and counting the number of drinks could help preserve your liver health.

Of course, it's wise to consume all good things in moderation. If you have trouble moderating your alcohol intake, it's best to just give it up completely and become a teetotaler. If you're already a teetotaler, there's no reason to start drinking red wine for your liver's sake. You can derive many of the same benefits from eating red or purple grapes or drinking (dark) grape juice.

There's another, hidden benefit of limiting your alcohol consumption: The effects on your weight. After slimming down and getting fit after having children, Jasmine, 40, had tried everything to lose the last 10 pounds of her excess body weight. She was working out daily for at least an hour, consuming a healthy diet, and watching her portions. Her lack of weight loss was a complete mystery and prompted her to call me one evening after a bad experience shopping for bathing suits. I asked her to send me a list of everything she ate for one week. Despite maintaining a great diet and exercising regularly, Jasmine was in the habit of drinking two martinis a night—a substantial calorie addition to her otherwise healthy diet. She gave up her martinis and dropped 10 pounds within ten weeks.

Your gut health Another little-known factor that affects your liver is the types of bacteria that colonize your gut. Simply put, an unhealthy

balance of bacteria in your gut is thought to harm the liver by promoting fat deposits on the liver, altering insulin sensitivity (which
can lead to NAFLD), and sparking the inflammatory cascade that can
damage the liver, among other mechanisms. Fortunately, you can
repopulate your gut with healthy bacteria by consuming probiotic-
containing foods and taking probiotic supplements (as you'll see in
Chapter 7). Intestinal permeability (a.k.a. leaky gut syndrome) is another emerging risk factor that's manageable. While you won't find
this term in standard medical textbooks—at least not yet, because
it's such a newly identified problem—the syndrome, which involves
the permeability of the intestines and their ability to keep toxic and
harmful bacteria from going outside the gut, is being pointed to as a
culprit in many chronic health conditions, including autoimmune disorders and fatty liver disease. Here's how it works: Ideally, when you
consume food, your body digests it thoroughly and is able to absorb
the nutrients fully. But if your gut is permeable, leakage may occur,
and instead of absorbing all the protein, fat, carbohydrate, vitamins,
and minerals from your food, some of those nutrients leak out of the
gut and into the bloodstream, causing inflammation in various parts
of the body, including the liver; toxins and food particles that aren't
digestible also can leak into the bloodstream. Determining whether
you have a leaky gut, however, may not be as straightforward as you
might think since symptoms often mimic (or precede) other digestive
conditions such as irritable bowel syndrome, Crohn's disease, and celiac disease. These symptoms can include bloating, gas, abdominal
cramping, food sensitivities, or even headaches and achy joints.

If you feel you may be suffering from a leaky gut, it's important
to find a physician who is up on the latest research on the syndrome;
your best bet is to ask your primary care physician for a referral to a
specialist in gastrointestinal diseases or a functional or integrative
medicine practitioner or to contact a nearby medical school. The doctor may initially put you on an elimination diet to assess if symptoms
go away or may even run an intestinal permeability test to determine
whether you have leaky gut.

The good news is, the dietary factors associated with healing a
leaky gut are similar to the same principles that are necessary for
a healthy liver: to take a break from drinking alcohol for at least

Believe it or not, the human gut is home to trillions of tiny organisms, including at least one thousand species of bacteria that can have a powerful impact on your health. You may be aware that the bacteria in your gut play a role in digestion, aiding your ability to digest certain foods or to fight certain bacterial infections (such as foodborne illnesses). As it turns out, these effects comprise just the tip of the glacier.

In recent years, groundbreaking research has shed light on the extent to which your gut microbiome (the community of bacteria that reside inside you) can influence your overall immune function and energy level, as well as your chances of becoming obese or depressed or developing cancer, diabetes, dementia, metabolic syndrome, or NAFLD. Specifically, the liver and the gut interact in myriad ways, through a connection known as the gut-liver axis. Strong evidence now links the gut microbiome and the integrity of the intestinal barrier function (particularly whether it has a strong epithelial lining) with the onset and progression of NAFLD.

Let's unravel these elements: While an excess of bad bacteria or an imbalance between good and bad bacteria in the gut is the first concern, the next is that the lining or integrity of the gut can become more permeable over time; increased permeability is commonly known as leaky gut syndrome. Picture the lining of your intestines as a long hose: As the lining gets worn down and develops tiny tears, it becomes more permeable; when this happens with your intestines, toxins and bad bacteria can slip out of the intestines and enter your bloodstream, causing a cascade of inflammatory effects throughout the body. This low-grade, systemic inflammation in turn increases the risk of developing type 2 diabetes, cardiovascular disease, NAFLD, and NASH. In other words, changes in the gut microbiome can play a role in the development and progression of gut barrier dysfunction, which can in turn lead to low-grade inflammation and liver damage.

The good news is, the composition of your diet can improve the state of your microbiome and your gut barrier integrity. Simply put, you can alter the bacteria in your gut by choosing foods that feed the good strains of bacteria and decrease the population of bad bacteria. The keys are to consume plenty of dietary fiber, prebiotics (foods that provide fuel for probiotics), and probiotics (foods that contain live bacteria and yeasts that are good for your health), and to keep your consumption of alcohol in the moderate zone. You'll find details on how to make your diet work optimally for your gut-liver axis in Chapter 7. Extensive use of antibiotics and nonsteroidal anti-inflammatory drugs (NSAIDs) can also compromise your gut-liver axis, as you'll see in the next chapter.

a month, to stop using nonsteroidal anti-inflammatory drugs (NSAIDs), such as aspirin and ibuprofen; to avoid sugar and artificially sweetened foods; and to adopt an anti-inflammatory diet that contains healthy fats found in fatty fish, nuts and seeds, as well as plenty of fruits and vegetables, legumes, spices, roots, whole soy foods, and unrefined whole grains. (You'll read more about this in Chapter 8.) You may also want to talk to your doctor about whether you'd benefit from taking probiotic (health-promoting bacteria) supplements and glutamine supplements. In Chapter 7 you'll read more about how to heal leaky gut and boost your liver health at the same time.

Viruses These are also under the umbrella of modifiable risk factors because you can take steps to avoid them. It's widely known that certain viruses, including many hepatitis infections, can cause liver inflammation and damage. The most common types of hepatitis infections are hepatitis A, B, and C. Hepatitis A is transmitted when a person consumes contaminated food or water (specifically, food or water that's tainted because a person infected with the virus didn't wash his or her hands properly before handling it). Hepatitis B is spread primarily through blood, semen, and other body fluids during sex or drug use with contaminated needles; it can also be passed from a mother to her baby at birth. Hepatitis C is spread through contaminated blood from infected needles from drug use and or dirty equipment used for tattoos. Before 1992, hepatitis C was also passed through blood transfusions and organ donations. Other viruses that can cause liver damage and even liver failure include Epstein-Barr virus, cytomegalovirus, SARS, parvovirus, severe influenza, and herpes simplex virus.

Adding insult to injury, when you already have one form of liver disease, being exposed to a liver-damaging virus or having liver-damaging lifestyle habits can do even more harm. In other words, there can be a cumulative effect. Henry's story is a good example of this. Henry, 67, was slightly overweight, worked long hours at a big law firm and was going through a divorce. The majority of his meals consisted of take-out food and his stress levels were through the roof.

Henry also had hepatitis C that was diagnosed when he was in his thirties and had always been well controlled with medication.

During a recent visit to his hepatologist, he found that his liver enzymes had gone up and this revelation, along with months of severe fatigue, is what prompted his visit to me to help him "clean up his diet." Henry and I decided on a plan that involved eliminating simple sugars, refined grains, and eating out. He also agreed to eat at least five servings of green leafy vegetables a day, and he started meditating to reduce stress and working out with a personal trainer four days a week. That was more than a year ago. Today Henry is eating right, managing his stress better, and exercising, and his liver enzymes have returned to a healthier level.

Metabolic syndrome This is another medical condition that plays a substantial role in liver health and contributes to the development of NAFLD and NASH. To refresh your memory: Metabolic syndrome is a constellation of risk factors for type 2 diabetes, stroke, and heart disease. It is diagnosed when someone has at least three of the following: elevated blood pressure (equal to or greater than 130 mm/hg systolic/85 mm/hg diastolic), insulin resistance or elevated fasting blood sugar (above 100 mg/dl), excess abdominal fat (a waist circumference greater than 40 inches for men, more than 35 inches for women), high triglycerides (150 mg/dl or higher) and/or low HDL (the "good") cholesterol levels (defined as less than 40 mg/dl in men, less than 50 mg/dl in women).

More than 50 million people in the United States are estimated to have metabolic syndrome, and 80 percent of them are likely to have NAFLD, as well. The syndrome stems largely from following a modern lifestyle—particularly, being overweight, consuming a poor diet, and being sedentary.

Fortunately, you have more control over the health of your liver than you may think you do because the number of modifiable risk factors for liver disorders far outnumbers those that aren't modifiable. Body weight, for example, is largely determined by how much food you consume and how much energy you expend; it's not all about genetic factors. In fact, even if you have a family history of obesity,

SLOW AND STEADY IS THE WAY TO GO

Since losing excess weight is essential to decrease NAFLD, you might think that the sooner you get those extra pounds off, the better. But it turns out that rapid weight loss can actually increase the risk of NAFLD in those who don't yet have it. When you lose weight quickly, there's often a sudden, dramatic release of pockets of toxic substances (particularly, organochlorines and polychlorinated biphenyls [PCBs], from environmental exposure) that have been stored in the liver; this surge of toxins causes liver enzymes to rise initially and strain the liver as a result. Plus, with rapid weight loss, a surge of fatty acids is released into the bloodstream as your fat cells shrink, and the liver can't cope with the deluge. It's almost as if the liver needs to have a chance to catch up to the weight change.

The good news is, NAFLD that's associated with rapid weight loss is usually temporary and is likely to subside as the weight loss slows or settles down. But if you continue dropping pounds at a rapid pace, NAFLD can worsen or lead to scarring. To sidestep this risk entirely, it's wise to stick with a gradual approach to weight loss, on the order of up to 2 pounds per week (as you'll see in Chapter 10).

research suggests that often it's our lifestyle choices that influence whether a gene will act against us and cause us to gain weight—or not. Eat the wrong foods (deep-fried items, for example) and you may encourage your genes to pack on excess weight, but feed your genes the right foods (such as fruits, vegetables, legumes, and healthy fats) and you may just tell those fat-accumulation genes to take a hike. The rate at which you burn calories varies from person to person, based on a variety of factors including the amount of lean muscle you have, genetic influences, your activity level, and more. But, in general, if you take in more calories than you actually use for fuel, that extra energy will get stored as fat.

Remember Terri? After a year on a slow, but sustainable weight-loss program that included cutting out sugar, incorporating more vegetables, healthy fats, and lean proteins, and reducing her overall carbohydrate consumption—a plan that's similar to the one in this book—Terri was able to slim down and get her BMI into the normal

range (under 25). Naturally, she was thrilled about her newly slim status, but even more exciting was the fact that she had more energy, felt
happier, and had achieved normal liver enzyme levels, a sign that she
had improved her liver health.

Ultimately, the best approach to protecting your liver and reducing your risk of developing liver diseases, such as NAFLD, is to keep
your weight in a healthy range (or lose excess weight if you need to)
and follow a wholesome, balanced diet. That means reducing your
consumption of fructose, other added sugars, and red meat; keeping
your fat intake in a healthy range; and limiting your alcohol consumption (and opting for red wine whenever possible). Chapters 9
and 10 contain specific plans to help with this; in the next chapter,
I'll address the risks of environmental exposures and chronic use of
certain medications. If you have any of the risk factors that were just
described, consider this a wake-up call that you need to swing into
action to protect your liver starting now. Improving your lifestyle
habits (the modifiable risk factors) can help you overcome or mitigate
many of the unmodifiable risk factors, such as having a genetic susceptibility to liver disorders. You'll find that if you take good care of
your liver, it really will take good care of you.

chapter 4

Everyday Toxins and Other Surprising Dangers from Modern Life

IN 2008, Emmy Award-winning actor Jeremy Piven left the Broadway production of the David Mamet play *Speed-the-Plow* after suffering from severe fatigue, weakness, dizziness, and nausea. The diagnosis: mercury toxicity from his twice-a-day sushi habit and from taking Chinese herbs to promote good health. Mercury is an element that's found throughout the environment, thanks in large part to industrial plants releasing the chemical into the water supply and air, and it is often absorbed in concentrated amounts by certain fish such as tuna and swordfish. Piven's mercury level was reportedly nearly six times the upper tolerable limit, which could have led to permanent damage to his brain, heart, kidney, lungs, and liver. He was fortunate: thanks to implementing dietary restrictions and taking key nutritional supplements, Piven seems to have made a full recovery.

In some ways, we live in a fairly toxic world, with harmful chemicals in our air and water, pesticides on our produce, antibiotics in our meat, contaminants in the fish we eat, and other potential hazards that can't be detected by the naked eye. To a large extent, our body does whatever it can to protect us from the potential harmful effects of these environmental factors—and all things considered, the liver does a masterful job of detoxifying our body on a regular basis. But some of us become overexposed to detrimental influences and/or our personal habits thwart our body's efforts to successfully handle damage control, and the liver (not to mention other organs) can't keep up with the challenges. That's when certain liver disorders can begin to appear.

High levels of mercury in the body are associated with a threefold increase in liver damage. High levels of lead and PCBs (short for polychlorinated biphenyl, a synthetic, organic chlorine compound) confer similar risks, and all three industrial chemicals may play a role in unexplained nonalcoholic fatty liver disease (NAFLD), according to the Integrated Medical Institute. In fact, a recently named phenomenon called toxicant-associated fatty liver disease (TAFLD) is similar in pathology to NAFLD and alcoholic fatty liver disease (AFLD) but considerably less common than these other diseases. TAFLD occurs in people who aren't obese and don't consume significant amounts of alcohol, but who have been exposed to high levels of environmental chemicals through food, water, and other means (if they work with or near industrial chemicals, for example). As with NAFLD and AFLD, TAFLD progresses slowly over several years and is largely asymptomatic until serious damage has been done.

During routine blood work as part of his annual checkup, John, 43, a married chemical engineer with a child in college, was found to have elevated liver enzyme levels. He was never a drinker or a drug user. He is lean with a BMI of 23 and he doesn't have diabetes, high blood pressure, cholesterol abnormalities, or any risk factors for liver disease, so the culprit behind the abnormal liver-enzyme readings was a mystery. John was referred to Dr. Hanouneh who decided to perform a liver biopsy, which showed a chemical type of liver injury. During a follow-up appointment and an in-depth discussion, it became apparent that at work John is exposed to monomeric vinyl chloride, a well-known chemical that's toxic to the liver.

Unfortunately, there isn't a specific treatment for chemical damage to the liver, except to avoid further exposure (which John was advised to do). Fortunately, his biopsy showed minimal scarring of the liver, so the hope is that his liver will repair itself given this vital organ's remarkable ability to heal and regenerate.

Typical Household Toxins

These unseen chemicals don't cut a direct path to the liver when they're absorbed. Their effects are sneaky and insidious. As it happens, exposure to high levels of pollutants, such as mercury and lead, can decrease antioxidant activity in the body (primarily by inhibiting functional enzymes and depleting levels of the essential amino acid glutamine, which is involved in protein metabolism, muscle preservation, gut function, and immune function) and affect proteins and enzymes in ways that disrupt normal liver function. Exposure to contaminants also may alter gene expression in the liver in ways that increase the risk of liver cancer. Complicating matters, obesity and fatty liver disease decrease the ability of antioxidants to fight against foreign invaders, such as mercury and lead: Once the body's antioxidant defenses are down, metabolism of these harmful substances is impaired (that is, the liver's detoxification power decreases), which in turn increases injury to the liver. Whether it's due to obesity, specific dietary factors, or exposure to environmental contaminants, cellular damage to the liver can put people at risk for liver damage—these are equal opportunity threats! Here are some of the biggest culprits:

Common household chemicals Some of these can be bad news for the liver, too. Research has found that when certain toxic chemicals are absorbed through the skin, eyes, mouth, or airways in excessive amounts, they can cause internal inflammation, mitochondrial dysfunction (an impairment of the cells' powerhouses to do their job), and oxidative stress. There's even a condition called toxic hepatitis, a form of liver inflammation that can occur when someone is exposed to high levels of chemical solvents, such as dimethylformamide (which is used in the production of fibers, adhesives, pesticides, and surface coatings) as well as tetrachloroethylene and trichloroethylene (both of which are used as degreasing products and spot-cleaning agents in dry cleaning).

Pesticides Organochlorine pesticides, which have been banned in the United States since the 1980s but still linger in the environment, have been linked with liver damage; these chemicals can make their way into our food supply through our waterways (in which case fatty fish can absorb them) and our soil (in which case they can end up in our fruits, vegetables, grains, and dairy products). Meanwhile, animal studies have found that Roundup, an herbicide that contains the chemical glyphosate and is widely used as a weed killer, can damage the liver by causing mitochondrial damage and by increasing oxidative stress in this vital organ. In 2015, the International Agency for Research on Cancer, the France-based research arm of the World Health Organization, labeled glyphosate, the main ingredient in Roundup, a "probable carcinogen."

Plastics In addition, we live in a highly plasticized world and bisphenol A (BPA), which is widely used in plastic water bottles and plastic food-storage containers, can harm the liver. In a 2012 study involving mice, researchers in Korea found that when the animals were administered doses of BPA below the level where no adverse effects have been observed for a period of five days, they still experienced mitochondrial dysfunction in the liver, which was associated with an increase in inflammation and oxidative stress—a detrimental double whammy!

How to Eliminate Risks

While most of us don't knowingly or intentionally expose ourselves to these potentially damaging chemicals, we all can take steps to avoid these hazards. And it doesn't have to be as complicated as you might think. Here's how you can do this on an everyday basis:

- Dry out your dry cleaning. Hang up dry-cleaned items outside your home to let the chemicals air out, and take off the plastic coverings before you put the items in your closet. Or find a dry cleaner that uses greener approaches to cleaning. Don't be fooled by dry cleaners that use the "organic" label, however: Even *dry cleaners* that use such solvents as perchloroethylene (PERC), which the Environmental Protection Agency has classified as "a probable human carcinogen," can claim to be organic. Your best bet is to ask questions about how clothes are cleaned. Safe, nontoxic approaches—such as wet cleaning and carbon dioxide cleaning—are available. Opting for washable clothing over those that need to be dry-cleaned can also reduce this risk.

- Clean up your home-cleaning products. At home, use organic or naturally derived cleaning solutions, especially for jobs that involve degreasing, removing oil from fabrics, or making something water repellent. In general, try to choose the least toxic products possible (hint: the fewer ingredients and the fewer ingredients you can't pronounce, the better). Keep in mind that solutions that are water-based are less harmful. Try to steer clear of products that contain the words DANGER, WARNING, or CAUTION, which often mean the item contains a substance that's harmful to human health.

- Organic does matter. Buy organic fruits and vegetables or purchase from a local farm (but only after asking about pesticide use). Thoroughly rinse all fruits and vegetables before cooking with them or eating them. Some fruits, such as waxed apples, should be peeled before they're consumed. Find out which fruits and vegetables are the highest and which are lowest in pesticide use and absorption by consulting the Environmental Working Group's "Dirty Dozen" and "Clean Fifteen" lists at http://www. ewg.org/foodnews/summary.php.

- Go for glass. Ditch plastic food storage containers and mixing bowls and opt for glass ones instead. If you can't eliminate plastic bottles and other plastic items from your home, buy only those with the recycle codes 1, 2, 4, 5, and 6 because these are unlikely to contain BPA. Use fewer canned foods (since the lining of the cans may contain BPA), and stick with more fresh or frozen choices.

- Make your home a shoe-free zone. Take off your shoes before you enter your home (and ask others to do so as well) to minimize the tracking in of harmful fertilizers, pesticides, and other chemicals.

- Round up the Roundup. Avoid using harmful chemicals on your lawn (or hire a green lawn-care company). Store any chemicals that are used to treat the grass and weeds in a secure, well-ventilated area.

- Replace old items with greener versions. It's not likely that you'll throw out your carpets, couches, and mattresses just because

**ENVIRONMENTAL WORKING GROUP'S
"DIRTY DOZEN" AND "CLEAN FIFTEEN"**

Dirty Dozen
- Strawberries
- Apples
- Nectarines
- Peaches
- Celery
- Grapes
- Cherries
- Spinach
- Tomatoes
- Sweet bell peppers
- Cherry tomatoes
- Cucumbers
- + Hot peppers
- + Kale and collard greens

www.ewg.org

Clean Fifteen
- Avocados
- Sweet corn
- Pineapples
- Cabbage
- Sweet peas, frozen
- Onions
- Asparagus
- Mangoes
- Papayas
- Kiwis
- Eggplants
- Honeydew melon
- Grapefruit
- Cantaloupe
- Cauliflower

they may contain chemicals. But when you're shopping for new furniture, it's wise to look for items that are free of phthalates (in wood varnishes and lacquers), flame retardants (used in foam and fabrics), volatile organic compounds (in plywood and particleboard), perfluorinated compounds (used in stain-resistant fabrics), and other potentially toxic chemicals. For tips on how to find chemical-free furniture, consult the Natural Resources Defense Council (www.nrdc.org) and the Environmental Working Group (www.ewg.org).

Risks We Expose Ourselves to Voluntarily

Besides taking steps to protect yourself and your loved ones from sneaky chemicals in the environment, it's important to pay attention to substances you choose to ingest that may be harmful to your liver and other organs.

Smoking This is a habit that 18 percent of adults, age eighteen and older, still choose to do in the United States, according to the Centers for Disease Control and Prevention. The leading cause of preventable disease and death, cigarette smoking accounts for more than 480,000 deaths every year. Even if it doesn't kill you, smoking can harm the liver in myriad ways.

Some studies have found that heavy smoking (defined as going through two or more packs per day) can damage the liver by increasing proinflammatory cytokines that are directly involved in damage to liver cells, by producing chemical substances that increase inflammation and scarring of liver tissue, and by reducing the capacity of red blood cells to carry oxygen, which can lead to the increased storage and absorption of iron, which can in turn result in oxidative stress to the liver cells. Whether smoking leads to an increased risk of NAFLD or accentuates the depositing of fat on the liver has been somewhat controversial. For example, in a 2010 study involving obese rats, researchers from Spain found that cigarette smoking causes oxidative stress and worsens the severity of NAFLD. More recently, an analysis of data from the Third National Health and Nutrition Examination Survey (NHANES III) found that smoking was not associated with the prevalence of NAFLD.

Long story short: We really don't know whether smoking increases the risk of fatty liver disease or accelerates the progression of the disease. But we do know that the nicotine and other chemicals from smoking are among the greatest toxins you can introduce into your body, so kicking the habit will benefit your health in numerous ways. For one thing, smoking increases the risk of heart attacks and strokes, which are by far the most common causes of death in people with fatty liver disease.

Medications Meanwhile, other substances that we ingest intentionally—ironically, to treat various health conditions or to improve our well-being—can harm the liver if too much of the wrong ones or if dangerous combinations are taken. On the drug front, some medications can directly injure the liver or lead to weight gain that can increase the risk of NAFLD; in other instances, the liver can transform certain drugs into chemicals that can harm this vital organ. This may seem counterintuitive, given the liver's crucial role in converting toxic chemicals into nontoxic ones—but, hey, it happens and more often than you might think.

Acetaminophen The best-known medication that can damage the liver is acetaminophen (Tylenol). In recent years, acetaminophen overdoses have grabbed headlines, as the phenomenon has become the leading cause of acute liver failure, according to the Food and Drug Administration. Each year, an estimated 78,000 people go to emergency rooms for intentional or accidental acetaminophen overdoses and 33,000 are hospitalized. Even before it progresses to the point of a medical emergency, acetaminophen overload is fairly common.

When taken in therapeutic doses, acetaminophen is safe, and animal studies suggest that more than 90 percent of a single dose is broken down into nontoxic metabolites—that is, as long as there is enough glutathione, an enormously important antioxidant present in the body. Sometimes referred to as "the master detoxifier," glutathione is a simple molecule that acts as a star player in the immune system, helping fight infections and prevent cancer, protecting cells from oxidative stress, attracting toxins and making them stick then sending them to be excreted from your body, and more. As long as sufficient glutathione is present, the liver is protected from injury. Overdoses of acetaminophen, whether it's a single large ingestion or overly high doses over a repeated period of time, can deplete glutathione stores in the liver, allowing injury to this organ to occur. Heavy drinkers and poorly nourished people are especially vulnerable to acetaminophen-induced liver toxicity because they have low levels of stored glutathione.

Not long ago, a 25-year-old man named Alex came to the Cleveland Clinic with a toothache. During a medical evaluation, the physician discovered that Alex had been taking large doses of over-the-counter acetaminophen along with a prescription acetaminophen-hydrocodone pain reliever for five days. Blood tests revealed that his liver enzyme levels were sky high—thirty-two times higher than normal for ALT (alanine aminotransferase), and fifty-eight times higher than the upper end of normal for AST (aspartate aminotransferase); elevated levels of these liver enzymes indicate inflammation or damage to the cells in the liver. Alex, a physical therapist who's married with one child, didn't have any risk factors for liver disease: he would drink no more than a couple of beers on the weekends; he had no history of intravenous drug use, tattoos, or blood transfusions; nor did he have diabetes, hypertension, or high cholesterol levels.

In his case, the elevated liver enzymes were clearly due to taking too much acetaminophen. This young man was lucky: His condition was caught before liver-related symptoms emerged and the condition became truly life threatening. He was treated with intravenous N-acetylcysteine, a medication that's used to treat acetaminophen overdose, and over the following week, his liver enzyme levels returned to the normal range.

Other drugs Besides acetaminophen, other drugs can harm the liver. These include **statins** (for cholesterol abnormalities), **antifungal drugs** (for fungal infections), **tamoxifen** (to treat breast cancer and prevent recurrence), **corticosteroids** (for autoimmune diseases or asthma), **certain antidepressants and antipsychotic drugs**, **birth control pills**, and some **oral hormone treatments**. Long-term use of some of these medications has been linked with abnormal liver-enzyme levels and sometimes an increased risk of developing fatty liver disease; however, it isn't clear whether the latter is due to a direct result of the medication's effect on the liver or a consequence of weight gain that's triggered by the medication (which occurs with many antidepressant or antipsychotic medications, in particular).

Sometimes, too, the effects are temporary and resolve on their own, as Adam, 54, a married ophthalmologist with two teenagers, discovered. He was found to have surprisingly high cholesterol levels, given that he was only mildly overweight (with a BMI of 28). Because he had a family history of high cholesterol and heart disease, Adam was placed on a low-fat, low-carb diet and he began jogging for twenty to forty minutes every day. Despite his losing 7 pounds (a major accomplishment!), his cholesterol improved only minimally so his primary care physician put him on a statin drug to reduce his cholesterol. When he began taking the medication, his liver-enzyme levels were normal, but they were mildly elevated at his three-month follow-up appointment. The results were thought to be due to the statins, an effect that's not unusual and often normalizes within a few months of treatment as the liver adapts to the medication. Adam was monitored closely with regular blood tests that eventually showed a complete normalization of his liver enzyme levels. As Dr. Hanouneh notes, it's rare that statins need to be discontinued because of abnormal liver-enzyme tests—but it can happen if the abnormalities don't resolve over time.

By contrast, long-term use of **corticosteroids**, especially in high doses, can result in enlargement and inflammation of the liver. Used to treat asthma, lupus, rheumatoid arthritis, inflammatory bowel disease, and many other medical conditions, these potent anti-inflammatory drugs also can trigger or worsen nonalcoholic steatohepatitis (NASH) or chronic viral hepatitis, such as chronic hepatitis B or C. Rest assured: If you're taking one of these medications on a continuous basis, your doctor will likely catch any liver enzyme abnormalities during your annual blood work; if you're taking a medicine that's known to be particularly toxic to the liver (such as certain antifungal drugs, or methotrexate, which is used to manage Crohn's disease or rheumatoid arthritis), your doctor will monitor your liver enzymes regularly during treatment.

Taken too often, a family of medications called **nonsteroidal anti-inflammatory drugs (NSAIDs)** can harm the liver directly and/or indirectly. Direct damage tends to be idiosyncratic—meaning, it's relatively rare and not dependent on dose—but it can happen and it can be transient or it can present as acute hepatitis (complete with fever, malaise, jaundice, and itching). Women and older adults are most vulnerable to this direct effect, as are people with chronic hepatitis C. In addition, frequent use of NSAIDs (including aspirin, ibuprofen, and the prescription drug celecoxib) can alter the bacterial composition of the gut microbiome, especially if these drugs are used in combination with proton-pump inhibitors (for gastroesophageal reflux disease, a.k.a. GERD) or antidepressants. As you learned in Chapter 3, the bacterial composition of the gut also can affect the liver's health and ability to function, thanks to communication along the gut-liver axis.

Supplements Many people typically take dietary supplements with the goal of improving or maintaining their health, but too much of the wrong vitamins, minerals, or herbs can cause severe liver injury: Too much vitamin A can be toxic to the liver, and excess iron may promote the formation of scar tissue in the liver and the risk of hemochromatosis (a genetic disorder involving excessive accumulation of iron in the body; see page 43) in those who are susceptible. Meanwhile, herbal supplements—including kava (often taken for anxiety), ephedra (for weight loss), skullcap (for anxiety or insomnia), yohimbe (for sexual arousal), and pennyroyal (for digestive disorders)—have been associated with acute liver failure, so your best bet is to avoid these entirely.

Even certain plants can be toxic to the liver. A couple of years ago, Edward, 63, went to the emergency room with a sudden case of severe nausea, vomiting, and abdominal pain. He hadn't traveled recently or been in close contact with sick people, so the reasons for his illness were mystifying. His blood tests showed abnormal liver function: Specifically, his levels of AST and ALT were ten times higher than the upper limits of the normal range. To try to get at the root of these abnormalities, Edward was screened for hepatitis A, B, and C—and all the tests yielded negative results. An ultrasound of his liver showed that it was slightly enlarged but otherwise most of the liver looked normal.

When Dr. Hanouneh questioned Edward, a father of three grown children, and his wife in greater detail, it became apparent that Edward had been eating wild mushrooms from his yard, something he claimed to have been doing throughout his life without any problem. Dr. Hanouneh and his team went to the patient's house to pick up mushroom samples for analysis and they discovered *Amanita phalloides* (commonly known as "the death cap," a deadly poisonous fungus) in the sample.

Over the next eighteen hours, Edward's condition deteriorated and he entered a state of liver failure. He also became highly confused and unable to breathe normally, so he was intubated and placed on a respirator. After being evaluated to see whether he was a candidate for liver transplantation, Edward was approved and listed as a priority for a transplant, given how critically ill he was. Fortunately, a match came up within 48 hours and he had a liver transplant without major postoperative complications. In fact, he recovered from surgery quite well. It's been two years since he had the transplant and results of his liver function tests are within normal limits, thanks in part to anti-rejection medicines. So far, Edward's story has had a happy ending, but not all patients with liver failure do.

The Liver's Distress Signals

Here's the unfortunate reality: Symptoms of liver disorders are often vague until the conditions become fairly severe. Someone with a liver disorder in the early stages might feel mildly tired, but let's face it: who *doesn't* feel tired these days? Given our collective tendency to cram as many activities into our waking hours as possible, a certain amount of fatigue is normal and understandable. So, feeling tired wouldn't automatically make you concerned about your liver health, whereas having your skin or the whites of your eyes turn yellow (jaundiced) might, as it should.

Although jaundice, which is caused by a buildup of bilirubin (a bile pigment) in the blood, is a telltale sign of some liver diseases—including hepatitis, cirrhosis, and liver cancer—it doesn't occur with others. In fact, most liver disorders, including NAFLD, don't cause noteworthy signs that unmistakably point to a problem with the liver, so people are often left in the dark about the presence of a liver disorder until it becomes fairly advanced (as in the case of NASH).

Among the more common symptoms of other liver disorders are itchy or overly sensitive skin; urine and stool changes (particularly, a darker urine and paler stool); abdominal tenderness and swelling; loss of appetite, nausea and/or vomiting; unexplained weight loss; a tendency to bruise easily; and fluid retention in the legs, ankles, and feet. In rare instances, more obvious symptoms, such as pain in the center or upper right part of the abdomen, and patchy, dark skin discolorations called acanthosis nigricans (usually on the neck or underarm area) are apparent, especially in kids, but these often indicate that insulin resistance is present, too. As liver diseases progress, a deep, persistent fatigue, muscle weakness, memory loss, and mental confusion may occur, as it did in Edward's case.

...n a liver problem isn't suspected until the results of blood tests for liver function present abnormal readings. The most basic tests, which are usually included in routine blood tests ordered by a physician, include those for the liver enzymes ALT and AST. Levels of these enzymes are reliable indicators of liver-cell injury and are helpful in recognizing liver diseases such as hepatitis. What's considered a normal level can vary from one laboratory to another, but often the normal range for AST is between 10 and 40 units per liter and a normal ALT level is between 7 and 56 units per liter. When levels get to be two to three times higher than the normal range, they're considered to be mildly elevated; the severity of the elevations and the degree of concern increase from there.

By that point, your liver's ability to detoxify substances, metabolize drugs and alcohol, remove the by-products that result from the breakdown of these substances, and clear bacteria from the bloodstream is somewhat compromised. Its ability to metabolize carbohydrates, protein, and fats and convert these macronutrients into forms of energy the body can readily use also may be somewhat under par. These are just a few of the reasons why it's important to catch liver problems in their early stages before substantial damage has been done.

If you have any symptoms of liver distress or a strong family history of liver disorders, it's wise to have blood tests to assess your overall liver function. Your doctor should include these automatically as part of routine blood tests but it doesn't hurt to check. If the results are out of whack, additional blood tests may be in order to look for specific liver problems, such as hepatitis, hemochromatosis, Wilson disease, or primary biliary cholangitis (a progressive disease caused by a buildup of bile, a fluid that helps with digestion, within the liver). When it comes to NAFLD or NASH, other liver conditions need to be ruled out to make the correct diagnosis.

Depending on the findings of various blood tests, an ultrasound, a CT (computed tomography) scan, or an MRI (magnetic resonance imaging) scan may be used to look for fatty deposits, scarring, or damage on the liver. Ultrasound scanning (a.k.a. sonography) produces

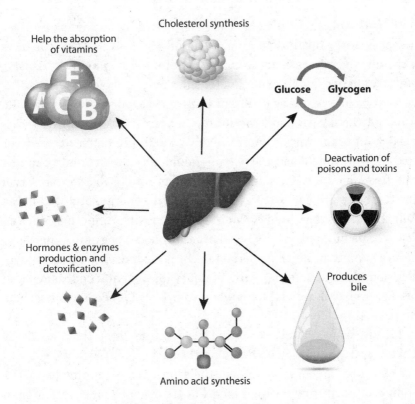

Functions of the liver. © Designua/Shutterstock

images of the inside of the body (in this case, the liver), using sound waves. CT scans are basically special X-rays that produce cross-sectional images of the body that appear on a computer. By contrast, MRIs use a large magnet and radio waves to look at organs, such as the liver. Each of these scans can help diagnose different disorders and diseases, but some are more effective than others.

In a 2004 study comparing the diagnostic accuracy of various abdominal imaging methods, researchers from the Medical University of South Carolina in Charleston found that MRI provides the most accurate diagnoses of liver and pancreatic diseases; ultrasound did the best job of diagnosing gallbladder disease, and CT scans and MRIs tied when it came to identifying kidney diseases. Here's the hitch: Ultrasound is much less expensive than CT scans and MRIs, which is why it's often prescribed first. MRI is the most expensive imaging tool of the three, but it's also the most accurate at diagnosing liver diseases. If the results of your ultrasound are equivocal or if you have a chronic liver disease and you're at risk for developing liver disease, you should discuss with your doctor whether you should have an MRI.

As you can see, many different hazards of modern living can take a toll on the health and functioning of your liver. When this indispensable organ can no longer remove waste products, bacteria, or toxins from your blood the way it should, or when its ability to metabolize macronutrients and convert them into usable forms of fuel for the body are compromised, your health, energy, and well-being will suffer. It's that simple. And if fatty deposits, inflammation, and scar tissue build up on this vital organ, you can begin to experience severe symptoms, such as persistent fatigue, muscle weakness, nausea, vomiting, abdominal pain, memory loss, mental confusion, and other worrisome signs. That's when your liver is sending out serious distress signals.

Ideally, you want to notice and heed subtle signs that your liver isn't operating the way it should on the early side. That way, you can see your doctor promptly and get the proper liver function tests, the right diagnosis, and optimal forms of treatment sooner rather than later. Just as it's much easier to turn around a small sailboat than a large cruise ship, the same thing is true of reversing a liver disorder in the early stages, compared to late-stage liver disease. This is an instance where timing matters enormously! An expedient diagnosis and early initiation of treatment can improve your chances of restoring your liver to a state of better health, which will have positive ripple effects on your entire body.

part two

Showing Your Liver a Little Love

chapter 5

Liver Love:
Basic Steps and Strategies

NOT LONG AGO, a woman named Barbara, 68, came to the Cleveland Clinic for an endoscopy to assess the varicose veins she had developed in her esophagus, a complication that's related to her liver cirrhosis. Barbara was significantly overweight, but not obese, and she had been diagnosed with nonalcoholic fatty liver disease (NAFLD) several years earlier. Neither she nor her husband, who had significantly elevated cholesterol and triglyceride levels, were drinkers, but they were a meat-and-potatoes kind of family (with large portions), and they didn't really know what a healthy diet looked like. Over the years, Barbara's fatty liver had turned into nonalcoholic steatohepatitis (NASH), then into cirrhosis of the liver. During a recent appointment, she asked, "Why did I get cirrhosis? Is this my fault?"

It was a heart-wrenching moment but a reasonable question. Still, casting blame doesn't do anyone any good, she was simply told that we should focus on how to improve her diet to take better care of her liver going forward. But the truth is Barbara hadn't been tending to her liver or her overall health the way she should have been.

She's hardly alone on that front. The good news is, it's rarely too late to turn the tables and start giving your liver the TLC it deserves and requires to stay healthy and in turn keep you healthy. You may find the prospect of doing things differently daunting—but don't despair! Chances are, you don't need to make a complete 180-degree turn in your lifestyle. For many people, making even small, focused changes to their habits and preventive strategies can add up to make a considerable difference to the health of their liver. These include:

· Limiting your alcohol intake

- Getting plenty of good-quality sleep on a regular basis
- Getting a grip on stress
- Minding your medicines
- Maintaining a healthy weight
- Having key blood tests
- Becoming a stickler for good hygiene
- Getting the right vaccines

Here's how to do it:

Limit your alcohol intake The link between someone's level of alcohol consumption and his or her risk of developing a liver disease varies from one person to another, but several factors can predict the person's vulnerability. If you have a family history of liver cirrhosis or alcohol-induced fatty liver disease, you may be especially susceptible to alcohol-related liver damage. If you carry a genetic variant that makes you prone to negative physiological reactions to alcohol (such as facial flushing, nausea, and rapid heartbeat), you also may be especially vulnerable.

As you saw in Chapter 3, factors that affect the development of alcohol-related liver injury include the amount, duration, and type of alcohol that's consumed; the person's drinking patterns; his or her sex and ethnicity; and associated risk factors that include obesity, iron overload disease (hemochromatosis), infection with viral hepatitis, and various genetic factors. In short, the more frequently people consume alcohol and the more they consume during each drinking occasion (especially if they engage in binge drinking, which is defined by the National Institute on Alcohol Abuse and Alcoholism as having five or more alcoholic beverages in a two-hour period for men, four or more for women), the more at risk they are for alcohol-related liver damage. This is especially true for women who have a family history of cirrhosis and people who are obese. In fact, research from the United Kingdom and Australia found that obese women who consume fifteen or more drinks per week have a five times higher risk of developing liver cirrhosis as do obese women who have a maximum of seven alcoholic beverages per week.

HOW MUCH DO YOU DRINK?

Approximately two-thirds of adults in the United States drink some alcohol, most in small or moderate amounts. A subgroup of drinkers, however, imbibes excessively, develops physical tolerance and withdrawal, and may be considered to have alcohol dependence. Another group—often referred to as "alcohol abusers" or "problem drinkers"—suffer from negative social and health consequences of drinking (such as unemployment, relationship problems, accidental injury, organ damage, and other ill effects). Binge drinking is the most common form of excessive alcohol use in the nation: One in six adults in the United States binge-drinks four times a month, consuming about eight drinks on each of those occasions, according to the Centers for Disease Control and Prevention. And research by Philip J. Cook, PhD, a professor at Duke University, found that the top 10 percent of drinkers in the United States consume close to seventy-four alcoholic beverages per week on average. (That's more than seven drinks per day!)

For those who have experienced adverse health or personal effects from drinking, abstinence is the best course of action. Abstinence has been shown to improve liver injury, reduce portal pressure and decrease the progression to cirrhosis, and improve survival for patients with alcohol-related liver disease. This improvement can be relatively rapid, and significant improvement is often seen in three months. (If you have trouble abstaining on your own, talk to your doctor about programs and/or medications that can help you quit drinking.)

Of course, you don't have to hit rock bottom or suffer negative repercussions from drinking to want to cut back. If you're concerned about how much or how frequently you're consuming alcohol, even though you haven't experienced adverse effects from drinking, it may be wise to reduce your consumption. Here are four good ways to do that:

- **Give yourself a limit**. Before you go out, decide how many servings of alcohol you'll allow yourself and stick with that maximum. Remember: Moderate drinking is defined as 2 drinks per day for men, 1 per day for women; and 1 drink is equal to 12 ounces of beer, 5 ounces of wine, or a shot (1.5 ounces) of spirits (a.k.a. hard alcohol).

- **Pace yourself.** Take small sips and do it slowly, and enjoy your cocktail. Putting down your drink between sips naturally helps you slow down (by breaking the automatic hand-to-mouth movement). Don't rush to have another one after finishing a drink; have a nonalcoholic beverage (such as club soda with lemon), take a break to chat or dance, or chew gum between drinks.
- **Take days off.** In general, try to have at least 2 alcohol-free days per week to give your body (and your liver) a break. After a night of overindulging, avoid alcohol for at least 48 hours.
- **Find new ways to socialize.** Go bowling or for a bike ride with friends. See a movie or take a yoga class. Or simply go to a party and have a nonalcoholic drink or alternate between the 2 beverages. You might be surprised that it doesn't matter what drink you have in hand, just having a glass of something—it doesn't need to be alcoholic—makes you feel part of the festivities. Remind yourself that the point of being there is to see people you know, meet new ones, and have a good time. Alcohol doesn't have to be part of the equation.

Get plenty of good-quality sleep on a regular basis Whether it's because of your overly hectic lifestyle or an underlying sleep disorder, getting insufficient shut-eye day after day can lead to liver dysfunction. It carries the added risk of wreaking havoc with your hormone levels (particularly ghrelin and leptin, which regulate appetite and feelings of fullness) in ways that may rev up your hunger and promote weight gain, which can also harm your liver.

Most adults need seven to nine hours of slumber per night. Here are some tips to make sleep a priority:

- Carve out enough time on a nightly basis (or near-nightly basis) to get the shut-eye you need to feel and function at your best.
- Establish a consistent sleep schedule by slipping under the covers and waking up at the same time every night and day.
- Vary your sleep schedule slightly on the weekends, but try to limit it to an hour in either direction at most; otherwise, you'll

disrupt your body's circadian (sleep-wake) rhythms and basically give yourself a modest case of jet lag.

It's not just the bedtime routine that can make a difference; here are some daytime tips to help you sleep better at night:

- During the day, spend time outside in natural light, even when the weather is overcast, to keep your body's internal clock ticking properly and help you maintain a healthy sleep-wake cycle.
- Getting some exercise during the day also can help set you up for a good night's sleep; try to finish vigorous workouts by late afternoon so that your body temperature, heart rate, and other bodily functions have plenty of time to drop before you turn in for the night.
- Be sure to steer clear of obvious stimulants (such as coffee, tea, and cigarettes) as well as sneaky ones (such as chocolate and soda) for 4 to 6 hours before you go to bed.
- While having a couple of glasses of wine or cocktails may make you sleepy initially, it can act as a stimulant after a few hours, leaving you vulnerable to microarousals or awakenings; this is another good reason to limit your alcohol consumption to a max of 1 or 2 drinks per day.

Sleep disorders If you have a sleep disorder, consult a sleep specialist so you can get it treated. Your liver is depending on it! After all, as you learned in Chapter 2, people with obstructive sleep apnea (OSA), a potentially serious condition in which someone repeatedly stops breathing, typically for ten to thirty seconds at a time, then starts again during sleep, have significantly higher levels of the liver enzymes ALT (alanine aminotransferase) and AST (aspartate aminotransferase), according to a 2015 study from Massachusetts General Hospital in Boston, and a substantial percentage of those with OSA have NASH. While the underlying reasons for the link aren't fully understood, they may have to do with metabolic factors—such as abdominal obesity and insulin resistance—that are associated with the development of fatty liver disease and are common among people with OSA. In another study from 2015, researchers from Taiwan found that the risk of liver disease—including NAFLD, cirrhosis, and hepatitis C—was more than five times higher among people with obstructive sleep apnea than among their peers who don't have the sleep disorder.

Get a grip on stress Letting stress get the upper hand can make you especially vulnerable to a variety of liver disorders, both directly and indirectly. If you're chronically stressed out, higher than normal levels of stress hormones (such as cortisol) will be coursing through your veins. These stress hormones can cause widespread inflammation throughout your body, including in the liver, where it can lead to slow but insidious damage, and they can promote the accumulation of fat in the abdomen, which has also been linked with an increased risk of developing NAFLD.

During the first nine months of his baby boy's life, Peter, 36, a software engineer for a financial company, and his wife were thrown into the sleep deprivation that's common among new parents. Adding insult to exhaustion, things at work were stressful and demanding and between the long hours Peter spent at his desk and the demands of a new baby, his exercise regimen fell by the wayside and he gained 20 pounds. To help relieve stress, he was drinking more than usual, often six to eight beers a day. He felt exhausted and frayed at the ends, which he attributed to lack of sleep and long hours at work, but his wife urged him to see a doctor. After lab tests showed elevated liver-enzyme levels, Peter had an ultrasound of his liver, which revealed severe infiltration of fat in this vital organ—most likely a result of the weight gain and excessive use of alcohol that stemmed from stress overload.

In a 2015 report, researchers from the University of Edinburgh in Scotland found that psychological distress (as in, symptoms of anxiety and depression) was linked with an increased risk of dying from liver disease: The primary mechanism seems to be inflammation, but the research also found that acute or chronic stress can lead to abnormalities in the body's central stress response system (officially known as the hypothalamic-pituitary-adrenal, or HPA, axis) and the sympathetic nervous system, which results in the release of proinflammatory factors in the liver and ultimately can lead to the development of NAFLD. In addition, the research noted that nonstop

TIPS FOR STRESS REDUCTION

While it may be your go-to, relying on junk food, alcohol, cigarettes, or the herb kava to ease your stress or tension is not the answer because these substances can have toxic effects on the liver. Instead, make it a priority to regularly practice wholesome stress-management techniques, mind-body interventions that relieve or ease your stress from the inside out, to support the health and vitality of your liver. Here are some "start small" tips to help minimize daily stress:

- Upgrade your time-management skills by prioritizing what needs to be done today and what can be deferred until tomorrow.
- Practice saying no to unnecessary requests, so you can save your time and energy for important activities and tasks.
- Delegate tasks that aren't essential for *you* to take on.
- Regularly perform relaxation techniques (such as meditation, hypnosis, acupuncture, or others) that dial down your body's response to stress.

Relaxation techniques really can make a difference, physiologically as well as psychologically. In fact, a 2015 study from the Republic of Korea found that a single session of a technique that combines meditation with special postures and abdominal breathing significantly reduces oxidative stress and levels of stress hormones (such as cortisol) in the body. Similarly, a 2015 study from China found that when nurses practiced yoga for fifty to sixty minutes after work three or more times per week for six months, their self-reported stress went down and their sleep quality improved. Various forms of meditation—including mindfulness meditation and self-compassion meditation—also have been found to reduce stress and anxiety.

Just do something healthy on a regular basis to prevent stress from flooding your body and your liver with the damaging effects of cortisol and accelerated wear and tear.

stress can lead to imbalances in blood levels of minerals, such as iron and copper, which can become toxic to the body and damaging to the liver if they build up and are not excreted properly.

Research also suggests that high anxiety can significantly decrease blood flow through the liver and trigger elevations of ALT levels, which can be associated with damage to liver cells. Moreover, studies have found that stress can exacerbate existing liver disease: in particular, many people who have hepatitis C report that a period of intense stress often precedes a flare-up of their symptoms.

Whatever the mechanisms may be, this much is crystal clear: Unbridled stress is harmful to your liver, just as it is to the rest of your body. Consider this reality yet another wake-up call that it's time to take steps to reduce and/or better manage stress in your life. To help yourself get a pulse on the sources of stress that get under your skin, how they affect you, and what you do to cope, use the Stress-Trigger Tracking Sheet in Appendix B, then resolve to develop better stress-reduction habits.

Mind your medicines As you saw in Chapter 4, it's important to try to avoid excessive use of medications (such as statins, corticosteroids, antifungal drugs, and acetaminophen, among others) that can harm your liver. If avoidance isn't an option, you'll want to have your liver enzymes tested at regular intervals (as determined by your doctor) to make sure these drugs aren't negatively impacting that organ. Don't let this important detail slip through the cracks! (If you have an older family member who is taking lots of medications, advocate on his or her behalf to make sure the physician regularly evaluates the state of his or her liver.)

Similarly, it's important to use caution with herbal and dietary supplements. Among the herbs that can be toxic to the liver when they're taken in high doses are black cohosh (often used to reduce hot flashes and other symptoms of menopause); green tea extract (when taken at high doses for weight loss); chaparral (used for joint pain and weight loss); and germander (found in some weight-loss products). Even everyday vitamins, when consumed in excess, can be toxic to the liver. Chronic overconsumption of vitamin A, for example, can damage the liver, leading to abnormal growth of liver cells and potentially scarring.

Maintain a healthy weight If your weight is in the healthy range (a body mass index below 25), you're in the right place as far as your

LIVER PURIFICATION PRODUCTS: ARE THEY WORTH SWALLOWING?

These days, you can find a surprising array of liver detoxification and liver purification products on the shelves of pharmacies and health-food stores. Given the hype surrounding these capsules, you might think these would be a wise investment in your liver's health and well-being. Before you shell out your hard-earned money for these products, you need to understand what they can and can't do for you.

First of all, it's important to know that supplements aren't required to gain approval by the Food and Drug Administration, as drugs are, before coming to market. So, with any supplement, there's no way to know whether the product actually contains what the label says it does.

As far as liver-detox products go, many of these contain various herbs (such as dandelion, burdock root, garlic, fenugreek, oregano, nettle leaf, milk thistle, and others) as well as vegetable starch and water. While most of these ingredients aren't likely to harm you, they aren't going to have any magical effects on your liver. There's limited evidence regarding the impact of individual ingredients on the liver and no research on the efficacy of these products as a whole. Nevertheless, if taking these supplements inspires you to improve your diet and take other lifestyle-related steps to protect your liver, there's nothing wrong with that. But no detox product can compensate for poor dietary and lifestyle choices.

Remember, too, these products aren't without their risks. I have seen people who have had unpleasant adverse reactions to seemingly harmless supplements, so there's no guarantee that they'll agree with you. There are potential risks and benefits with any supplements but less is known about herbal ones, so you're taking your chances with them.

Bottom line: There is no magic bullet or singular supplement that can reset your liver health. If you do choose to take supplements to protect your overall health, be sure to do your research and find a reputable brand. If you are taking any medications, check with your doctor to find out whether there are specific supplements you should avoid, to protect yourself from potentially dangerous interactions.

liver is concerned. If you're overweight, slimming down can help protect your liver and potentially even reverse certain liver disorders. Researchers from Saint Louis University and Brooke Army Medical Center found that when overweight and obese people with NASH achieved a weight loss of at least 9 percent, they essentially reversed the damage their liver had experienced previously. A slow and steady rate of weight loss is the way to go, so you can sustain it and protect your liver's well-being. Remember: Rapid weight loss can actually increase the risk of NAFLD. A 2013 study from Iran found that when people with NAFLD followed a diet with a daily reduction of 500 to 1,000 calories—with 55 percent of those calories from carbohydrates, 15 percent from protein, and 30 percent from fat—for six months, they lost at least 5 percent of their body weight and gained significant reductions in their liver enzyme levels.

Have key blood tests Among the measures that can keep tabs on your liver health are blood levels of the liver enzymes ALT and AST, which may be part of the annual blood work that's ordered by your doctor (ask because if they're not, you should request these tests specifically). If your liver enzyme levels are elevated, but you don't have any worrisome symptoms, the first step is to have the test repeated in short order to confirm the results. If the results of the second test are still abnormal, your doctor should evaluate the extent of the elevation. A minor elevation (less than twice the normal value) may be of no clinical importance if the following disorders have been ruled out: Alcohol abuse, a medication side effect, chronic hepatitis B or C, steatosis, autoimmune hepatitis, hemochromatosis, Wilson disease, alpha 1-antitrypsin deficiency (an inherited disorder in which the body does not make enough of a protein that protects the liver and lungs from damage), celiac disease, inherited disorders of muscle metabolism, acquired muscle diseases, or extremely strenuous exercise (such as running marathons).

Depending on your ALT and AST readings and your personal risk factors, other blood tests might be recommended including ALP (alkaline phosphatase), another enzyme found in the liver as well as the bile ducts, and GGT (gamma-glutamyl transpeptidase), an enzyme found in the liver, bile ducts, and pancreas. Elevated levels of any of these may signal damage to or malfunctioning of the liver and/or bile ducts. But there are circumstances in which elevations in certain liver enzyme levels are physiologically normal; for example, ALP levels are naturally increased in healthy women during the third trimester of pregnancy. So, the evaluation of someone with an isolated elevation of ALT or AST is different from that for a patient with an isolated elevation of ALP or GGT; the approach needs to be personalized, in other words. (If your doctor isn't comfortable proceeding with an evaluation, ask for a referral to a hepatologist.)

By contrast, low blood levels of the proteins globulin, albumin, or prothrombin may indicate some degree of liver damage. And elevated levels of bilirubin (a brownish, yellowish pigment found in bile) may indicate different types of liver problems, such as hepatitis and drug toxicity. Keep an eye on the health of your liver by asking your physician to review the results of your blood tests with you and pay attention to where these liver-related enzymes and proteins fall on the spectrum of abnormal to normal; if any of these measures seems out of whack, ask your doctor why this might be and whether you should have follow-up tests.

Be a stickler for good hygiene Most of us don't think about proper hand-washing and other hygienic habits in terms of our liver health—but we should, because it's a smart way to steer clear of viruses (such as hepatitis A) that can harm the liver. Recently, a friend of mine was diagnosed with hepatitis A after suffering from severe nausea, blood in her urine, and fatigue. She had absolutely no idea how she got it: She hadn't traveled internationally; she didn't know anyone with the disease, and she doesn't drink alcohol or use drugs. Initially, how she caught the infection was a bit of a mystery. Within weeks, however, a hepatitis A outbreak was identified in the community and all the cases, including my friend's, stemmed from eating at the same restaurant. Clearly, the hepatitis A was a foodborne illness that likely came from a member of the kitchen staff not washing his or her hands properly. Hepatitis A is very contagious—you can catch it from eating contaminated food or touching a doorknob or an elevator button that was recently touched by someone who carries the virus (who happened to go to the bathroom but didn't wash his or her hands afterward), then rubbing your eyes or nose.

The lesson here: Wash your hands thoroughly and frequently (lathering up like a surgeon for at least twenty seconds each time) and carry an alcohol-based hand sanitizer with you. Also, since some forms of hepatitis stem from contaminated foods and beverages, my personal policy is to steer clear of restaurants that have been cited for foodborne illnesses in the past.

Get the right vaccines Vaccines are available that protect the liver from certain forms of hepatitis. Most people who have a form of liver disease should be vaccinated against hepatitis A and hepatitis B; both vaccines are safe and effective. After the series of either vaccine, you gain long-term protection from these liver-damaging diseases.

Hepatitis A is often caught from consuming contaminated food or water. The hepatitis A vaccine consists of two shots, with the second dose given six to eighteen months after the first; it is recommended for all children, for travelers to certain countries, and for other people who are at high risk for infection with the virus.

Hepatitis B is spread through contact with blood or other bodily fluids from an infected person. The hepatitis B vaccine is usually given as three intramuscular injections, the second and third administered one and six months after the first; it is now given to all children and recommended for adults who are considered at risk for hepatitis B (because they have more than one sexual partner, have a partner who is infected with hepatitis B, or have diabetes or chronic kidney or liver disease, for example). Practicing safe sex by using latex condoms can help protect you from hepatitis B and C, as well (note: there is no vaccine for hepatitis C).

Giving your liver the TLC it needs and deserves can be as simple as practicing these key steps; if you do so, this vital organ will return the favor in spades by protecting you from life-threatening illnesses. Peter, the software engineer/new father, achieved this by following a low-carb, low-sugar diet, cutting back on alcohol, and jogging for thirty minutes every other day, which eased his stress. Within six months, he lost 10 pounds, gained more energy—and his liver enzyme levels had completely normalized.

In the chapters that follow, you will learn more about how to manage your weight, make smart dietary decisions, and exercise wisely for the sake of your liver (and the rest of your body). Don't worry: This isn't a matter of reinventing the wheel or giving your lifestyle a complete overhaul. Many of these changes are easier to make than you may think. And once you start making these lifestyle shifts, you'll find that they're easier to stick with than you may have thought. Often, getting started is half the battle. With a nod to Sir Isaac Newton, just as a body in motion tends to stay in motion, establishing healthy lifestyle habits can quickly become a self-perpetuating prophecy as you see how simple they are to implement and how good you feel.

chapter 6

Move It:
The Protective Role
of Exercise

N OT LONG AGO, Rebecca, a 46-year-old librarian and divorced
mother of a teenage girl, was referred to the Cleveland Clinic's
liver clinic because she had abnormal liver enzymes. Her AST (aspartate aminotransferase) and ALT (alanine aminotransferase) levels
were two to three times the upper limit of normal, and an abdominal ultrasound indicated that she had fatty liver disease. Because
her screening tests for hepatitis B and C yielded negative results,
because Rebecca was a light drinker (who consumed a maximum of
two glasses of wine on the weekends), and because she had no family
history of chronic liver disease, the source of her fatty liver disease
became readily apparent: For most of her life, Rebecca had been obese
and her body mass index (BMI) was around 36. When she came to the
clinic, she had recently been diagnosed with type 2 diabetes, and her
triglyceride level was high (at 210 mg/dl) and her HDL (the "good")
cholesterol level was low (25 mg/dl). This combination of factors—a
BMI in the obese zone, type 2 diabetes, high triglycerides, and low
HDL—point to metabolic syndrome, a significant risk factor for nonalcoholic fatty liver disease (NAFLD).

   To improve her liver condition, Rebecca was referred for diet and
exercise counseling. She was placed on a health-promoting Mediterranean diet (you'll learn more about this diet in the next chapter) and
an exercise program that consisted of two to three forty-five-minute
sessions per week over twelve weeks. For her workouts, Rebecca chose
to do interval training on the treadmill—alternating bouts of jogging
with periods of walking. After twelve weeks, Rebecca returned to the
clinic for follow-up: she had lost 10 pounds, which reduced her BMI

slightly, but improved her liver enzyme levels dramatically; her AST level was back to normal, and her ALT level was elevated by just a few digits, not by a factor of 2 or 3 as it had been before she started the diet and exercise program.

When it comes to managing your body weight, you probably realize that it helps if you move your body regularly if you want to lose excess pounds. As I often tell patients, it's difficult to lose excess weight and sustain the weight loss if you're not willing to get regular physical activity. There are several reasons. For one thing, physical activity helps you burn extra calories while you're exercising as well as for several hours afterward (this is often called the afterburn effect—a.k.a. excess postexercise oxygen consumption, or EPOC, for short). That's right—you can continue burning calories at a faster rate even after your workout ends!

For another thing, when people lose weight, it's never 100 percent body fat; they lose lean muscle mass, too. Even when you're resting or doing ordinary activities (such as cooking, writing, or driving, but *not* exercising), pound for pound, muscle tissue burns considerably more calories than fat tissue does. So, if you lose a considerable amount of muscle mass, rather than mostly fat mass when you diet, your metabolism will slow down somewhat, which will make it that much harder to keep the weight off. Plus, a consistent exercise regimen doesn't just make you look better on the outside; it improves the way you look inside, too! Simply put, exercise is good for the appearance of your liver (and the way it functions), just as it is for your other internal organs.

Widely known for boosting cardiovascular health, regular aerobic exercise also reduces your risk of developing type 2 diabetes, hypertension, breast and colon cancer, depression, osteoporosis, and sneaky inflammation in the body. Over time, it leads to increased stamina, stronger muscles, improved immune function, and better weight control. Meanwhile, weight-bearing exercise and strength-training workouts build and protect your bone mass, reducing your risk of osteoporosis. Now, for the big surprise: Regular physical activity, independent of weight loss, is also good for your liver for a variety of reasons. Indeed, exercise is truly powerful medicine.

Giving Your Liver a Healthy Workout

The latest research suggests that people who engage in regular physical activity—including aerobic exercise and resistance exercise—have a significantly lower risk of developing NAFLD. Numerous studies also show that getting plenty of exercise is essential when it comes to increasing insulin sensitivity and facilitating loss of excess weight, which can in turn heal damage to the liver. Since fatty liver is often referred to as the hepatic (liver) expression of metabolic syndrome, and metabolic syndrome includes obesity and insulin resistance, getting more exercise may help reduce the risk of developing fatty liver and help in the fight to reverse it as well.

The truth is, insulin resistance and the presence of fat on the liver tend to go together like Bert and Ernie, Simon and Garfunkel, Abbott and Costello. It's hard to imagine one without the other. Insulin resistance is directly tied to an increase in glucose levels in the blood, as well as a rise in circulating fatty acids, which can damage the liver directly. In other words, the state of insulin resistance essentially helps maintain fat on the liver.

Exercise is part of the solution: Because exercise reduces insulin resistance, it helps prevent the buildup of fat on the liver or undermine its ability to stay there. Plus, exercise increases the oxidative capacity of muscle cells and increases the muscles' ability to use fat as energy, thus preventing excess fat from being stored in the liver. And a 2006 study from India found that regular moderate intensity aerobic exercise helps normalize ALT levels and reduce AST levels in people who have nonalcoholic steatohepatitis (NASH).

Even if you are overweight and/or already have NAFLD, it isn't too late to start reaping the benefits of moving more. A 2015 study from the University of Sydney in Australia found that aerobic exercise of various intensities and doses—whether it's 60 minutes of low to moderate intensity exercise four times per week, 45 minutes of high intensity exercise three times per week, or 45 minutes of low to moderate intensity exercise three days per week—reduced liver fat comparably among people who are overweight or obese even when they didn't lose significant amounts of weight. In other words, just doing any physical activity will help your liver. Another study from the University of Sydney, in 2009, found that after obese people did four weeks of aerobic cycling, they reduced fat tissue volume by 12 percent and triglycerides (another form of fat) in their liver by 21 percent. Meanwhile, in a recent study at the University of Tsukuba in Japan, 169 obese, middle-aged men with NAFLD participated in a twelve-week weight reduction program. Those who did at least 250 minutes of moderate to vigorous physical activity per week improved the state of their liver significantly, primarily by reducing inflammation, oxidative stress, and the presence of fat on their liver. Granted, 250 minutes of exercise per week is a lot for many people—equal to five fifty-minute workouts per week—but even those who exercised for 150 minutes per week upgraded their liver status.

It's Not Just About Body Weight

How does exercise improve liver health even when people don't lose weight? Physical activity influences chemical reactions that happen in the liver. When sedentary people begin doing aerobic exercise or resistance training regularly, they experience significant reductions in the accumulation of liver fat and abdominal fat, increased fat oxidation, and improved insulin sensitivity. Regular exercise also improves the efficiency of ATP (adenosine triphosphate) synthesis and its utilization; as a result, the transport of chemical energy within cells is improved, which helps all your muscles and organs function better. Exercise also seems to influence the diversity of gut microbiota, which may have beneficial influences throughout the gastrointestinal system, which may in turn have a positive ripple effect on the liver. And even though the previously mentioned study from Japan found that the weight-loss results associated with participating in a twelve-week exercise program were disappointing compared to a restricted-diet intervention, obese, middle-aged men with liver-function abnormalities who did the exercise training gained significant improvements in their liver enzyme levels, insulin resistance, and markers of inflammation and oxidative stress.

It's not just people with obesity-related liver diseases who can benefit from regular exercise. Even people whose weight is in the normal

WHEN EXERCISE COULD BE RISKY

By the time NASH or another liver disease progresses to cirrhosis, exercise may become problematic. For one thing, people with cirrhosis often show a reduced tolerance to exercise and have trouble sticking with it to the point where they would reach their peak aerobic capacity. This is partly because their cirrhosis-related symptoms—fatigue, physical deconditioning, insulin resistance, reduced liver function on a cellular level, and decreased cardio-pulmonary function, among others—interfere with their ability to work out, changes that can lead to reduced muscle mass and reduced strength over time.

range can. A 2014 study from Saudi Arabia found that after patients with chronic hepatitis C engaged in forty minutes of moderate intensity aerobic exercise (in this case, on a treadmill) three times per week for three months, they experienced a significant decrease in their liver enzyme levels—including ALT, AST, GGT (gamma-glutamyl transpeptidase), and others—as well as a significant boost in their psychological well-being. While it's widely known that regular exercise helps protect against breast cancer, colon cancer, and prostate cancer, whether the same can be said for liver cancer remains to be definitively determined. But there is some suggestion that this may be the case. For example, a 2013 study from Germany found that middle-aged adults who engaged in twenty minutes or more of vigorous physical activity at least five times per week had a 44 percent decreased risk of developing hepatocellular carcinoma (the most common form of liver cancer in adults) over the subsequent ten years, compared to their inactive peers. A 2015 study from the University of Berne in Switzerland found that regular exercise has a positive effect on the progression of liver cancer in mice that have NASH. Specifically, exercise reduced the growth of abnormal cells and induced apoptosis (cellular suicide) among abnormal cells.

In addition to aerobic exercise, resistance training is also good for your liver. A 2011 study from the United Kingdom found that after sedentary adults with NAFLD performed eight weeks of resistance training, they experienced a 13 percent decrease in fat on their liver, even though their body weight and percentage of body fat didn't change.

A 2014 study from Israel found that after patients with NAFLD did forty minutes of resistance training, three times a week (including three sets of eight to twelve reps of leg presses, chest presses, seated rows, lat pull-downs, and other exercises), they experienced a significant drop in their liver fat and other favorable changes in their body composition, even though they didn't lose weight. Resistance training can bring about other liver-related benefits, as well. For example, in patients with progressive liver disease, resistance exercise can help offset the muscle wasting that often occurs when they approach the point of needing a liver transplant.

All Movement Counts—as Does Consistency

As far as your liver is concerned, every bit of physical activity counts. That's why hepatologists (liver doctors) agree that regular exercise is a critical component for managing and potentially reversing NAFLD—and for keeping a healthy liver in optimal working condition and preventing problems from occurring. Ultimately, consistency is key: While taking a break from exercise for a week doesn't appear to hamper its benefits, longer interruptions (on the order of, say, four weeks) causes a deterioration of overall metabolic health and liver health, according to research in animals. The optimal approach for your liver's sake and your overall health is to do a steady combination of aerobic activity and resistance (or weight) training; this will help reduce fat on the liver, as well as improve fat oxidation in the body and blood sugar control. Think of it this way: the combo of aerobic exercise and resistance training is like delivering a one-two punch to excess fat on the liver.

Plus, regular physical activity can help relieve stress, improve sleep, boost mood (even alleviating depression and anxiety), and enhance your overall sense of well-being. So, moving more will help you feel better 24/7 and have the energy you need to make other healthy adjustments to your lifestyle.

Your Exercise Rx

For general health, the current recommendation is for adults to get at least 150 minutes of moderate intensity aerobic exercise each week—which comes down to 30 minutes a day, five days per week—as well as doing strength-training exercises at least two days per week. The aerobic part of the equation can be fulfilled with brisk walking, jogging or running, swimming, cycling, taking an aerobics class (such as step aerobics, kickboxing, or Zumba) or using a cardio machine at the gym (such as the elliptical trainer, a rowing machine, the treadmill, or the stair-climber). For the record, "moderate intensity" means that your heart rate and breathing rate increase but you can still speak in complete sentences; if it becomes too difficult to talk, you've crossed the line into vigorous exercise, and if you can talk so easily that you can sing, you're not working hard enough (it's light intensity, in other words).

Besides protecting your liver, boosting your cardiovascular fitness will help safeguard your overall health for longer. As proof, consider this: Women with the highest level of cardiorespiratory fitness at midlife have a 43 percent lower risk of developing heart disease, diabetes, chronic obstructive pulmonary disease, kidney disease, and other chronic conditions over the next twenty-six years than their less-fit peers do, according to 2012 research from the Cooper Institute in Dallas. That's a tremendous payoff!

When it comes to strength training (a.k.a. resistance training), you'll want to target all the major muscle groups in your shoulders, chest, back, arms, abdomen, hips, and legs—by using free weights, weight machines, your own body weight (as in push-ups and the plank), or a combination of these different approaches. In addition to protecting your liver, you'll be building muscle strength, muscle mass (but not bulk), and muscular endurance and revving up your metabolism, which can help you shed excess weight and burn body fat faster. It doesn't take as much of a time investment as you may think it does: Research from Southern Illinois University found that when overweight adults did one set of resistance training exercises—which took only fifteen minutes!—their resting energy expenditure (a.k.a. their calorie-burning rate) was elevated for seventy-two hours after the workout, just as much as when they did three sets of exercises. Doing resistance training will also help you counteract the progressive age-related loss of muscle mass that occurs to everyone (a condition called sarcopenia), a decline that begins in the thirties.

When you put the pieces together, here's what your weekly workout schedule might look like, whether or not you want to lose weight:

MONDAY: Swim or exercise on a cardio machine (such as a treadmill, elliptical machine, stair-climber, or stationary bike) for 30 minutes.

TUESDAY: Walk briskly for 20 minutes plus do a strength-training workout.

WEDNESDAY: Take an indoor cycling, Zumba, or step aerobics class for 45 minutes.

THURSDAY: Engage in brisk walking for 20 minutes plus do a strength-training workout.

FRIDAY: Work out on a cardio machine for 30 minutes.

SATURDAY: Rest.

SUNDAY: Go bike riding, hiking, or play tennis for at least 30 minutes.

(NOTE: This exercise Rx is *in addition to* making an effort to move more often throughout the day, perhaps by walking to a friend's house or on errands instead of driving, or taking the stairs instead of the elevator whenever possible.)

If you've been inactive or sedentary until now, start your new exercise regimen slowly so your body has a chance to adjust and work up to the length or intensity of the recommended workouts. You can also divvy up your exercise sessions and go for two fifteen-minute bike rides or walks, rather than doing a thirty-minute workout. Remember: Every bit of movement counts! You'll be doing your body and mind a great service just by moving more than you have been. Pay attention to the feel-good benefits you derive from increasing your physical activity—whether it's a boost in mood or energy, improved sleep, less stress, a brighter complexion, or something else—and you'll help yourself get hooked on getting and staying fit.

The Forgotten Fitness Factor

As part of a well-rounded fitness program, it's also wise to take time to stretch after your workouts. You can seize opportunities throughout

the day—while working at your desk or watching TV, for example—
to do some simple stretches. This is especially important, as you
get older, because as the decades go by, we all tend to lose flexibility
(which is sometimes called "the forgotten fitness factor"). The physiological reasons for this change: As you get older, the water content
of your tendons, the tissues that attach your muscles to your bones,
decreases, making your tendons stiffer and less able to withstand
stress; meanwhile, your ligaments, the connective tissues that connect bones to other bones, become less elastic, thus reducing your
flexibility. It's not just a matter of being able to touch your toes (or
not): Losing flexibility can set you up to injure yourself in everyday
activities, such as when you bend down to pick something up off the
floor. The good news is you can improve your flexibility with consistent effort. A 2015 study from Wayne State University in Detroit found
that when sedentary adults did yoga or a stretching-strengthening
regimen three times a week for eight weeks, they gained significant
improvements in their flexibility, mobility, balance, and strength—all
of which are considered measures of functional fitness.

Stretching Your Limits
Yoga offers the added benefit of providing specific perks to your
liver. In a 2014 study published in the *European Scientific Journal*, researchers who examined the effects of one and a half months of yoga
therapy on adults between the ages of twenty and fifty found that
those who developed the yoga habit experienced decreases in their
ALP (alkaline phosphatas e) levels and they lost weight. A 2015 study
from India found that when alcoholics participated in an intense
yoga program that involved practicing the mind-body discipline for
ninety minutes per day for thirty days, their blood levels of the liver
enzymes ALT and ALP dropped considerably.

What's more, practicing yoga can help you manage your eating
habits and your weight. A 2009 study from the University of Washington in Seattle found that the regular practice of yoga improves
people's ability to practice mindful eating (which involves slowing
down, being aware of the nourishing and enjoyable properties of food,
recognizing and honoring your physical hunger and signs of satiety,

and the like); by contrast, neither walking nor another type of moderate intensity exercise regimen enhanced participants' mindful eating scores. Plus, yoga's mindfulness component can help relieve your stress, improve your sleep, and help you feel and function better around the clock.

Meanwhile, certain yoga poses are believed to be particularly beneficial for the liver, according to the *Yoga Journal*, because they stimulate digestion, aid the detoxification process, and enhance overall health. Yoga classes are now available in many gyms from regular chains to YMCAs as well as at boutique studios—for everyone from beginners to hot yoga devotees—and include everything from gentle yoga for relaxation to yoga for pain relief or pregnancy health; if you want to exercise at home, you could invest in a yoga DVD (or two).

Here are four yoga moves that yoga experts believe to be especially good for your liver:

Wide-Legged Forward Fold in Chair
Face Forward Twist
Seated Side Twist in the Chair
Child's Pose in the Chair

These poses help improve the function and overall health of your liver by enabling a gentle massage and stimulation, which results in an increase in blood flow to the liver.

These movements are simple enough to practice at home on a daily basis. You'll need a sturdy, armless chair and it's probably best if you are wearing loose, comfortable clothing. Keep in mind: Yoga should never be painful. When you do these stretches or hold these poses, listen to your body and only stretch to the point of mild tension. Remember to breathe fully to gain maximal benefits from the movements. You can practice these poses daily, anytime or anyplace.

Wide-Legged Forward Fold in a Chair

Sit at the front edge of a sturdy, armless chair while lengthening your spine and lifting your heart. Your feet are flat on the floor, your knees are bent and aligned over your ankles, your toes and knees are pointed forward. Widen your legs into a comfortable V position with your ankles directly under your knees. Make sure your knees and toes are pointed in the same direction. Place your hands on the tops of your thighs. Inhale and allow your breath to fill your rib cage and your belly to expand for a deep breath. Lengthen the crown of your head toward the ceiling while extending your spine tall. Exhale and send your belly button toward your spine as you gradually fold forward, hinging at the hip and

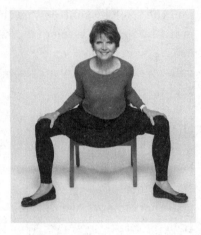

Wide-legged forward fold in a chair.
Reprinted with permission, Cleveland Clinic Center for Medical Art & Photography © 2016

maintaining straight alignment of your spine, neck, and head. Hold for one to two breaths or for what is comfortable. Return to the tall, seated position. Repeat two to three times.

Face Forward Twist in a Chair

Sit at the front edge of a sturdy, armless chair while lengthening your spine and lifting your heart. Your feet are flat on the floor, your knees are bent and aligned over your ankles, your toes and knees are pointed forward. Rest your hands on the tops of your thighs. Inhale and allow your breath to fill your rib cage and your belly to expand for a deep breath. Lengthen the crown of your head toward the ceiling while extending the spine tall. Exhale and bring your belly button toward your spine as you reach your right hand toward the

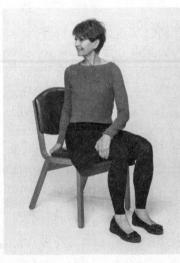

Face forward easy spinal twist in a chair.
Reprinted with permission, Cleveland Clinic Center for Medical Art & Photography © 2016

back of the chair and move your left hand onto your right thigh. Gently twist your whole upper torso toward the right. Allow your shoulders to stay soft and low, away from your ears. Hold the position here for one to two breaths or for what is comfortable. Return to the forward-facing position. Once again, take a few deep breaths, allowing your breath to fill your rib cage and your belly to expand. Lengthen the crown of your head toward the ceiling while extending your spine tall and upward. On your next exhale, bring your belly button toward your spine as you reach your left hand toward the back of the chair and move your right hand onto your left thigh. Gently twist your whole upper torso toward the left. Allow your shoulders to stay soft and low, away from your ears. Hold this position for one to two breaths or for what is comfortable. Return to the forward-facing position.

Seated Side Twist in a Chair

Sit at the right side of a sturdy, armless chair while lengthening your spine and lifting your heart. Your feet are flat on the floor, your knees are bent and aligned over your ankles, your toes and knees are pointed forward. Rest your hands on the tops of your thighs. Inhale and allow your breath to fill your rib cage and your belly to expand for a deep breath. Lengthen the crown of your head toward the ceiling while extending your spine tall and up. Exhale and bring your belly button toward your spine as you reach both hands to the top

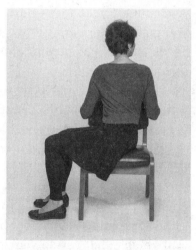

Seated spinal twist from the side of a chair. Reprinted with permission, Cleveland Clinic Center for Medical Art & Photography © 2016

edge of the chair back while gently turning your whole upper torso in a straight, tall line toward the right. Allow your shoulders to stay soft and low, away from your ears. Hold this position for one to two breaths or for what is comfortable. Release back to your starting position. Once again take a few deep breaths allowing the breath to fill your rib cage and your belly to expand. Check that your spine is still tall and your heart lifted. Now move your entire body over to sit at the left side of the chair. On your next exhale, bring your belly button toward your spine as you reach both hands to the top edge of the chair back while gently turning the whole upper torso in a straight, tall line toward the left. Allow your shoulders to stay soft and low, away from your ears. Hold this position for one to two breaths or for what is comfortable. Return to your starting position.

Child's Pose in a Chair

Sit at the front edge of a sturdy, armless chair while lengthening your spine and lifting your heart. Your feet are flat on the floor, your knees are bent and aligned over your ankles, your toes and knees are pointed forward. Rest your hands on the tops of your thighs. Inhale and allow the breath to fill your rib cage and your belly to expand for a deep breath. Lengthen the crown of your head toward the ceiling while extending your spine tall. Exhale and bring your belly button toward your spine as you

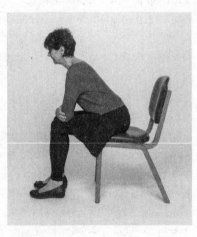

Child's pose in a chair. Reprinted with permission, Cleveland Clinic Center for Medical Art & Photography © 2016

gradually curl forward over your thighs. Allow your spine to soften while supporting your upper body with your hands or forearms on your thighs and resting your rib cage on your forearms, hands, or lap. Your head and neck are relaxed with your chin pointing toward your chest. Rest here for one to two breaths or for what is comfortable. Return to the tall, seated position. Repeat two to three times.

Now that you have the scoop on how and why aerobic exercise and resistance training can improve the shape of your liver, it's time to start thinking about how you can create a workout plan that works for you. Use the suggested weekly schedule on page 93 to build your own routine. Be adventurous and try different forms of exercise in different settings, and with various friends, neighbors, and other acquaintances, to see what appeals and what feels comfortable to you. If you've basically been as still as a statue until now, embark on your new exercise program in a gradual fashion, increasing the intensity, duration, and frequency of your workouts as your body adjusts and gets stronger. Remember: You want your workouts to feel somewhat challenging but also fairly energizing and manageable so that you can stick with them for the long haul and make them a habit. That's when your liver will really show its gratitude.

chapter 7

Liver-Friendly Eating Strategies

A FEW YEARS AGO, Kathryn came to see me because she wanted to lose weight. Although she had been slim in her teens and twenties, once a husband, three kids, a stressful nursing job, and "organized chaos" at home came along, her weight skyrocketed. After years of yo-yo dieting, she weighed more than 200 pounds. What's more, her lab results—particularly, her fasting blood sugar and lipid (cholesterol) levels—pointed toward a major case of metabolic syndrome, which, as you've learned, can take a toll on the liver. As a nurse, she knew about the cardiovascular risks associated with metabolic syndrome, but she was unaware that it could damage her liver, too. When I discussed this with her, Kathryn's motivation to lose the excess weight soared because, as a nurse, she understood all too well how important her liver is for her health and her survival.

One of the most common questions people have when they come to see me is: "What's the best diet?" It's a simple question with a complicated answer that depends partly on their personal goals. Whether they want to lose weight or gain muscle, improve their bone mass or heart health, or achieve another health-related milestone, there isn't a one-size-fits-all plan that works for everyone's needs. But there are some dietary patterns that apply to numerous health-boosting aspirations, including protecting the well-being and functioning of the liver. You've undoubtedly heard the maxim "Eat food. Not too much. Mostly plants," from Michael Pollan's book *In Defense of Food: An Eater's Manifesto.* Well, it's a mantra your liver will love, too!

Go Mediterranean

Long purported to be one of the healthiest eating patterns on the planet, the Mediterranean diet, which is what I recommended for

Kathryn (and Rebecca, whom you met in the previous chapter), ad-
heres to many of these principles. It consists of a high intake of fruits
and vegetables, whole grains, legumes, healthy fats (especially from
nuts, seeds, and olive oil), fish and seafood, and moderate amounts
of wine and dairy products. People who adhere to the diet tend to be
healthier and weigh less than those who follow the standard American diet (SAD) or what I like to call "the Western disaster" given its
detrimental effects on our health.

The Mediterranean diet is a perfect approach for reversing metabolic syndrome and liver conditions for several reasons: It lacks proinflammatory foods (such as simple sugars, high-fructose corn syrup,
sugar-sweetened beverages, refined or stripped carbohydrates, and
most saturated fats and trans fats) that harm the liver and various
aspects of cardiovascular health (including blood sugar levels, cholesterol levels, and blood vessel function). In addition, it lacks large
amounts of red meat, which is significant because consuming lots of
foods that are high in heme iron (beef, veal, lamb, pork, and other red
meats) can damage the liver by creating an overload of iron stores;
this is especially true for people who have a hereditary susceptibility
to iron overload or who are at risk for hemochromatosis, as noted in
Chapter 2.

Meanwhile, the Mediterranean diet contains foods that help regulate blood sugar levels and promote lipid control, which is significant
because reducing risk factors for cardiovascular disease and diabetes
tend to go hand in hand with boosting liver health. The mechanisms
for all three diseases really are *that* entwined! Following the Mediterranean diet can also increase antioxidant levels in your blood,
which will help your entire body, including your liver, fight oxidative
stress and damaging, low-grade inflammation. It's also a plan that's
sustainable because it's tasty, satisfying, and easy to follow since it
doesn't rely on the dreaded calorie-counting techniques that cause
so many people to throw in the towel when it comes to trying to lose
weight, in particular.

Like Kathryn, patients who have followed a Mediterranean-style
diet have often seen dramatic changes in their blood sugar and
lipid levels, their C-reactive protein level (a marker of internal

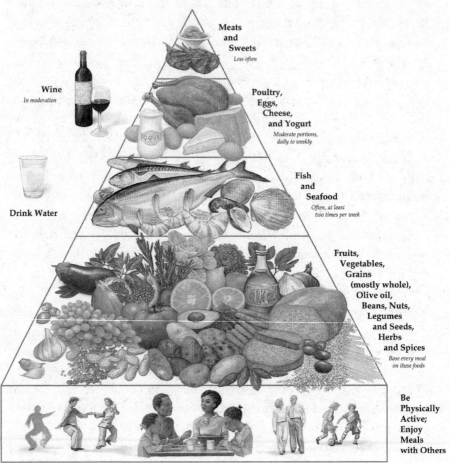

Mediterranean diet pyramid. © 2009 Oldways Preservation & Exchange Trust, www.oldwayspt.org.

inflammation)—and many of those who were overweight have lost at least 10 percent of their body weight, a benefit that's associated with the reversal of nonalcoholic fatty liver disease (NAFLD). A 2015 review of the research on the association between dietary intake and fatty liver disease found that a "Mediterranean diet intervention resulted in a significant decrease in liver fat content over six weeks." Similarly, a 2015 study from Italy found that when overweight people with NAFLD followed the Mediterranean diet for six months, they experienced dramatic changes in the fat content in their liver. For many people, whether their liver fat content decreases in six weeks or six months with the adoption of the Mediterranean diet, it's a change worth making and keeping for the sake of their liver and their overall health.

Go Low GI

Low-carb diets (a.k.a. a low–glycemic index lifestyle) can also enhance liver health, mainly by improving insulin resistance. The glycemic index (GI) measures how fast a carbohydrate-containing food raises blood sugar, compared to other foods: Foods with a low GI value (55 or lower) are digested, absorbed, and metabolized more slowly, which leads to a lower and slower rise in blood sugar and insulin levels. By contrast, foods with a medium GI value (56 to 69) and those with a high GI value (70 or more) cause blood sugar levels to rise rapidly. On a basic level, it's widely known that high-GI foods stimulate the production of insulin, which in turn promotes fat deposits especially in the midsection and increases fat accumulation in the liver as well.

Foods that have low glycemic effects—such as whole grains, legumes, vegetables, many fruits (when consumed in their natural, whole form, not as juice!), and healthful oils—tend to elevate blood sugar levels slowly after they are consumed. This means they help keep your blood sugar and insulin levels relatively stable over time and help prevent that postmeal blood-sugar roller-coaster ride that high glycemic foods can put you on. A low-glycemic plan omits starchy, sugary foods (such as cakes, cookies, and other baked goods), white rice, white pasta, and white potatoes, which have high GI levels and lead to a rapid spike in blood sugar and insulin levels. This is significant because, as you've already seen, the mismanagement of insulin inside the body plays a starring role in the development of NAFLD.

For more information on the low-GI diet, visit glycemicindex.com.

When insulin resistance enters the picture, a low-carb diet can come to the rescue by easing the strain on the liver. In fact, a small study at the University of Texas Southwestern Medical Center at Dallas found that when obese people with NAFLD cut their carb intake to

A QUICK RECAP OF THE CONNECTIONS

Researchers have found that as the obesity rate and the diabetes rate have soared in the United States, so has the incidence of NAFLD—and it's no mystery as to why: Insulin resistance occurs as a result of obesity, especially the apple-shaped (abdominal) pattern of obesity. When people have insulin resistance, the body produces insulin but it doesn't use it effectively, which causes glucose to build up in the blood instead of being absorbed by the cells.

Here's where the liver comes in: That excess blood sugar then heads to the liver to be processed and stored as glycogen, a form of future fuel for the body. (You might think of your liver as that extra fridge you keep in the garage—you know, the one where you store more food for the future.) If too much blood sugar floods the liver, your liver is forced to work overtime, triglyceride levels rise in the blood, and fatty deposits can develop on the liver. That's when your hardest working organ really takes a hit, as the formation of free radicals occurs, inflammatory factors creep up, and oxidative stress (a process in which unstable oxygen molecules damage cell membranes) starts taking a toll on the liver. It's a harmful triple whammy, indeed!

less than 20 grams per day for two weeks, they experienced a 42 percent reduction in liver fat. This was a significantly greater decrease in liver fat than what was achieved by obese people with NAFLD who simply cut their calorie intake.

If you want to stick with a lower-GI diet, consume high-fiber whole foods, which take longer to digest, such as legumes, nuts, intact whole grains, and vegetables throughout the day. Eating proteins on their own has no impact on blood sugar, but adding them into meals can help keep blood sugar levels under control. I often tell my patients to create "competition" for digestion when they eat foods that are higher in simple sugars: Pair an apple with no-added-sugar almond or peanut butter; eat pineapple chunks with a piece of cheese or mix them into yogurt; or have farro with half a chicken breast. In all three of these instances, the carbohydrates will compete with either protein or (healthy) fat to be digested, which leads to a slower rise in blood sugar.

Monica, 43, a case manager at a small community hospital who lives with her 14-year-old son, gained a significant amount of weight after getting divorced five years ago. She blamed the weight gain on the stress associated with the divorce and her sedentary desk job. When she went to see her primary care physician for her annual checkup, Monica's lab results showed abnormal liver enzyme levels. She doesn't drink alcohol heavily, nor does she use recreational drugs—but her BMI was 41 (significantly obese). An ultrasound showed diffuse fatty infiltration of her liver.

She was referred to a dietitian who recommended that she follow a low-GI diet that included lean protein in every meal, plus healthy carbohydrates (such as legumes, sweet potatoes, and quinoa) and healthy fats (such as extra-virgin olive oil, nuts, and seeds). A coffee lover, Monica was encouraged to continue her java habit but only with dark coffee, no cream or sugar (to reduce it to a low-GI beverage). Because her vitamin D level was low—and since low vitamin D status is associated with rapid progression of fatty liver disease—Monica was advised to take vitamin D replacement capsules daily. She was also advised to increase her physical activity level and aim for twelve thousand steps a day. Within six months, she lost 12 pounds and her liver enzymes normalized completely; so did her triglyceride levels, which had previously been mildly elevated.

Liver Health Superstars

While the overall pattern of your diet or your macronutrient intake can affect the health of your liver, it's also important to be detail-oriented by paying attention to your diet at the micro level—whether you go Mediterranean, low-GI, or with another eating plan. The reality is specific ingredients and food components can promote liver health, whether or not you have NAFLD, and these elements are essential parts of any healthful diet. These include foods that are rich in the following:

Phytochemicals These plant-based compounds, found in fruits, vegetables, nuts, and whole grains, have health-promoting properties in the body that may help prevent cancer, heart disease, and other

Fat gets a bad rap, but the truth is, dietary fats provide plenty of benefits to your body. They help you stay full for longer and assist in the absorption of fat-soluble vitamins (such as A, E, D, and K), and they help make food taste good. But not all fats are created equal.

For example, trans fats, which are found in some meats, dairy products, and processed foods, can wreak havoc on your blood lipids and ultimately your liver. The only way to tell if a packaged food contains trans fats is to read the nutrition label (if you see the phrase "partially hydrogenated oil" in the ingredients list, that's your tipoff and your cue to put the product back on the shelf). To reduce your risk of heart disease, I also recommend avoiding saturated fats, such as palm oil, palm kernel oil, and cottonseed oil. (Coconut oil, a plant-based saturated fat, can be used in small amounts for cooking or baking.)

Here's why the dietary details matter so much when it comes to fats: While it's known that obesity is a major risk factor for fatty liver disease, not everyone who is overweight or obese develops NAFLD—and in the past we haven't understood why this is the case. A 2015 study by researchers at the Medical University of South Carolina has shed light on this: The researchers fed two groups of mice a high-fat diet—one group consumed a diet high in saturated fat; the other, a diet high in unsaturated fat. Both groups became obese, but only the mice on the saturated diet developed liver inflammation and nonalcoholic steatohepatitis (NASH). When the researchers investigated further, they found that higher levels of a particular lipid molecule (called sphingosine-1-phosphate, or SIP, for short) caused inflammation in the liver; previous studies have found that excess saturated fat in the diet increases SIP levels. Connect the dots and it becomes clear why some obese people develop NASH—it's the saturated fat in their diet that's largely to blame.

For healthier fats, focus on getting plenty of monounsaturated fats (in avocados, olive oil, nuts, and seeds) and polyunsaturated omega-3 fatty acids. Your heart and your liver will appreciate the switch enormously. Remember, though, that a gram of fat has more calories than a gram of protein or carbohydrates does, so it's best to consume even healthy fats in moderation to keep your calorie consumption (and your weight) under good control.

life-threatening conditions. Indoles, lycopene, lignans, resveratrol, anthocyanins, and quercetin are among the bioactive compounds that are particularly beneficial to the liver, which is why you'll find them in the diet plans in Chapters 9 and 10. In fact, anthocyanins (found in the skins of blackberries, elderberries, raspberries, black grapes, and eggplant) help prevent fat accumulation and inflammation in the liver and counteract oxidative stress in the liver, according to a 2013 review of research on the subject. A phytochemical called quercetin, which is a flavonoid found in citrus fruits, apples, onions, parsley, olive oil, grapes, dark cherries, and dark berries, has been found to inhibit hepatitis C infection. And a 2015 study from China found that high doses of quercetin can alleviate the liver damage (especially due to fat accumulation) that's associated with consuming a high-fat diet. As noted in Chapter 5, supplements aren't subjected to testing and approval by the Food and Drug Administration (FDA) before they come to market, so I recommend consuming these beneficial compounds from foods—especially colorful fruits and vegetables—rather than from pills.

Coffee Java lovers can take comfort in the fact that regular consumption of the brew is associated with a decreased risk for type 2 diabetes, heart disease, stroke, gallstone disease, Parkinson's disease, and others, as well as a lower risk of overall premature mortality. Now there's a new benefit to add to the roster: Lower levels of ALT (alanine aminotransferase), AST (aspartate aminotransferase), and GGT (gamma-glutamyl transpeptidase), even among those with excessive alcohol intake, obesity, a smoking habit, and/or chronic viral hepatitis. Moreover, an analysis of four continuous cycles of the National Health and Nutrition Examination Survey (NHANES), a dietary intake questionnaire collected by the National Center for Health Statistics of the Centers for Disease Control and Prevention, revealed that caffeine intake was independently associated with a decreased risk of developing NAFLD. In a 2005 analysis of two prospective cohort studies, researchers from Japan found a significant inverse relationship between coffee consumption and the risk of liver cancer:

Compared to non-coffee-drinkers, java consumers who drank one or more cups daily had a 42 percent lower risk.

Since coffee is composed of hundreds of different substances, it's impossible to pinpoint which ones are responsible for these beneficial effects, and it may be that multiple compounds have synergistic effects (such as strong antioxidant properties *and* anticarcinogenic effects) that protect the liver. Whether you prefer your coffee black or with milk is up to you, but it's best to consume filtered coffee, which is largely free of oily substances called cafestol and kahweol that are known to raise cholesterol.

Omega-3 fatty acids Salmon, tuna, walnuts, flaxseeds and chia seeds, and other sources of these polyunsaturated fatty acids are essential for heart health and brain health, among other body functions. Because omega-3 fatty acids help improve blood lipid levels and lower inflammatory factors in your body, they are beneficial to the liver, as well. In fact, new research from Oregon State University found that an omega-3 fatty acid called DHA (docosahexaenoic acid) could have significant value in the prevention of fatty liver disease. Moreover, deficiencies in blood levels of omega-3 fatty acids have been shown to be a direct risk factor for the progression of NAFLD. A large multi-center study investigating the use of another omega-3 fatty acid, EPA (eicosapentanoic acid) to treat NASH is now under way in the United States.

Fiber There are two different types of fiber—soluble and insoluble—and each has distinct benefits to overall health. Soluble fiber, which is contained in foods that swell when they're placed in liquids (think: oats, beans, lentils, and ground or milled flaxseeds), can help reduce cholesterol levels and the overall risk of heart disease, and it's an important factor in maintaining a healthy gut, too. On the other hand, insoluble fibers, which are found in nuts, bran, brown rice, and the skins of fruits, add bulk and speed up the passage of food through the gastrointestinal tract. Both types of fiber are good for the liver: A 2007 study from Brazil found that when people with NAFLD took 10 grams of soluble fiber (in supplement form) each day for three months, their elevated liver enzymes decreased and they saw improvements in their BMI, waist circumference, insulin resistance, and cholesterol levels, too. Research has also found that getting enough dietary fiber is associated with a lower risk of developing type 2 diabetes (including insulin resistance), lower cholesterol and triglyceride levels, and better weight control—all of which may reduce the risk of developing liver problems as well.

Probiotics Good bacteria play a substantial role in promoting a healthy gut—and there's a positive carryover effect for the liver, due in part to the close interaction between the gastrointestinal tract and the liver. (Some researchers even use the phrase the *gut-liver axis* when referring to how bacteria in the gut might affect the liver and play a protective role against chronic liver damage, as you saw in Chapters 3 and 4.) In fact, alterations in the microbiota (the community of microbes, especially bacteria, that resides inside you) have been found in people with NAFLD, cirrhosis of the liver, and alcohol-related liver disease. The good news: Research suggests that restoring a healthy internal bacterial environment through the consumption of probiotics (health-promoting bacteria that naturally occur in certain foods) and prebiotics (nondigestible fiber compounds that stimulate the growth of probiotics) can have a beneficial effect on NAFLD, among other liver conditions. When it comes to liver health, probiotics also help reduce levels of low-grade inflammation and bacterial translocation (a.k.a. leaky gut syndrome, see pages 50-51). Consider this yet another good reason to stock up on yogurt, kefir, and other fermented foods, such as miso, kimchi, tempeh, and sauerkraut—or to take probiotic supplements.

A few years ago, Janice, a married woman in her mid-30s, came to see me because she had been suffering from digestive distress—including alternating bouts of diarrhea, constipation, abdominal cramping and bloating, gas, and random stomach pain—as well as headaches for several years. Slightly overweight (her BMI was 28), Janice also wanted to slim down. After tests found that she was sensitive to gluten and casein, Janice cut out whole wheat bread, which she had been consuming at every meal, and all dairy products. Within a few weeks, her symptoms improved, but not quite as much as we'd hoped they would, so we added probiotic supplements and another supplement with a broad array of digestive enzymes to her regimen to help her reduce gas and better absorb nutrients. After taking the probiotics for a month, Janice was headache-free and her digestive symptoms had improved dramatically. By improving her gastrointestinal function, she undoubtedly did her liver a huge favor, as well, since these organ systems are so intricately connected. An added benefit: Janice lost 5 pounds.

Soy proteins Soy often gets a bad rap because of its estrogenic properties, but a diet rich in whole soy sources (rather than processed ones) can have numerous beneficial health effects, including on the liver. Research has found, for example, that the bioactive compounds in soy (namely, isoflavones) can prevent and treat NAFLD by modulating fat metabolism and altering gene expression in the liver in ways that improve fatty acid oxidation in the liver. The net effect: a decrease in fat accumulation in the liver. Soy isoflavones also have been found to decrease inflammatory factors and improve glucose tolerance. The best sources of soy come in whole food forms, such as tofu, edamame, tempeh, and miso, not from soy chips or soy-containing energy bars (as the ingredient soy protein isolate).

Spices Besides adding taste bud-tickling flavor to your meals, such spices as turmeric, curry powder, and chile pepper (curcumin, the active compound found in turmeric, and capsaicin, the compound found in chile peppers that give them their spicy kick, are not themselves spices), ginger, and fenugreek seeds can help promote liver health. This is largely through their antioxidant properties, but in some cases also through their anti-inflammatory powers, their ability to alter gene expression, and/or their enhancement of detoxification enzymes. For example, a laboratory study published in the July 2014 issue of *Gut* found that curcumin inhibited the entry of hepatitis C virus particles into liver cells, and a 2013 study from China found that curcumin prevented the growth of liver cancer cells in a laboratory setting. Meanwhile, a 2013 study from Taiwan found that feeding essential ginger oil on a daily basis to mice with alcoholic fatty liver disease (AFLD) helped protect their liver from damage due to the disease. And 2011 research from Japan found that consuming fenugreek seeds inhibited fat accumulation in the liver in rats that consumed a high-fat, high-sugar diet.

Green tea While concentrated infusions of green tea extract, which are often found in popular weight-loss supplements, are problematic (because in large quantities they've been implicated as a potential cause of acute liver failure), drinking green tea in moderation is safe and may even be beneficial to the liver. There's even some evidence, according to a 2008 review of the medical literature in the journal *Liver International*, that when consumed in moderation, green tea may decrease the risk of liver disease, especially liver cancer. The perks may come from the polyphenols in green tea, which have been shown to reduce DNA damage and decrease blood lipid concentrations. The catechins in green tea also may help with the treatment of viral hepatitis. My suggestion is to steer clear of supplements that contain green tea extracts and to stick with the real stuff—a soothing brew of green tea, hot or cold.

Vitamin E An antioxidant that protects the body from damage caused by free radicals, vitamin E can help safeguard the liver's health if you consume adequate amounts of this fat-soluble vitamin in your diet. Research suggests that vitamin E can help lower elevated liver enzymes, prevent the progression of NAFLD, and reduce the development of scar tissue on the liver. It's best to get this vitamin from food, not supplements, so stock up on vegetable oils, nuts, seeds, whole grains, and eggs, for their vitamin E content.

One important note: Too much of this fat-soluble vitamin can be problematic, especially for people who have heart disease or take blood thinners. What's more, some reviews of the medical literature have reported an increase in all-cause mortality with high doses of vitamin E (while others failed to confirm such an association), and a 2011 study from the Cleveland Clinic found that taking 400 IU of vitamin E per day significantly increased the risk of prostate cancer among healthy men. These are additional reasons why it's best to get this vitamin through food rather than supplements.

Choline An essential B vitamin the body needs for normal physiological functions, including many that take place in the liver, choline plays a major role in the metabolism of VLDL (very low-density lipoprotein, the form in which triglycerides are secreted from the liver). When choline stores are low in the body, fat can build up in the liver, which in turn impairs normal mitochondrial function and reduces fatty acid oxidation, and gut bacteria may be altered in detrimental ways. *This is bad news all the way around!* What's more, several studies have shown that choline deficiencies may help set the stage for NAFLD and liver cancer, whereas having a higher choline level may help prevent these diseases. Choline is found in eggs, shellfish, poultry, peanuts, wheat germ, and whole soy foods.

Besides supporting the overall health and functioning of your liver, these superstars you've just read about can help reverse or stop the progression of NAFLD. But the benefits don't stop there. This dietary approach also can have positive ripple effects by helping you lose excess weight, preventing or reversing type 2 diabetes, and lowering your risks of heart disease and stroke, among other diseases. In other words, by following a diet that relies primarily on whole grains, vegetables, fruits, legumes, nuts, and healthy oils (such as olive oil) with smaller portions of fish and seafood, dairy foods, and occasional servings of red meat—you'll hit the bull's-eye for how to eat for optimal health, including the well-being of the liver. This way, you'll get plenty of health-promoting phytochemicals, anti-inflammatory omega-3 fatty acids, gut-protective probiotics, and other food compounds that will help you feel and function at your best.

The next chapter offers some strategies for making these changes. In Part 3, you'll find two liver-protective diets that rely on this nutritional approach. Depending on whether you want to lose weight or maintain your current weight, you can choose the one that appeals to you and suits your needs. Either way, if you stick with the delicious health-promoting foods in your chosen plan, before you know it, you'll fuel your body with high-quality energy, you'll safeguard your liver health, and you'll thrill your taste buds, too.

While I'm generally not a fan of taking supplements for the reasons I've already described, there are two that may be worth taking for your liver's sake.

Vitamin D In the United States, vitamin D deficiency is more common than many people think—the overall prevalence is 42 percent, with the highest rates seen in African Americans, followed by Hispanics. Besides being associated with a host of health problems (such as heart disease, diabetes, multiple sclerosis, depression, and certain forms of cancer), vitamin D deficiency has been linked with a worsening of various liver diseases, including cirrhosis, hepatitis C, and cholestatic chronic liver diseases (which involve a reduction or stoppage of bile flow).

In this case, restoring what's missing may help improve liver health: A 2014 study from Iran found that when people with NAFLD were given high doses of vitamin D supplements every two weeks for four months, they experienced significant decreases in their levels of a compound that reflects harmful free radical activity, as well as considerable reductions in their hs-CRP levels (a marker of systemic inflammation). And a 2013 study from Japan found that giving patients with chronic hepatitis C infection supplements of vitamin D_3, a potent optimizer of the body's immune response, could improve their response to antiviral therapy and other therapies for the infection.

Probiotic supplements While the research on the use of probiotics for various liver diseases has yielded mixed results, there is some evidence that taking these supplements can be beneficial. For example, a 2005 study from Italy found that treating people with NAFLD or alcoholic liver cirrhosis with the probiotic VSL#3 led to improvements in liver function tests and a reduction in proinflammatory cytokines. A 2011 study from Spain found that when people with NAFLD took a tablet containing the probiotics Lactobacillus bulgaricus and Streptococcus thermophilus every day for three months, their levels of the liver enzymes ALT, AST, and GGT decreased considerably. Other studies have found that taking probiotics can prevent a decline in brain function that can occur as a result of severe liver disease (a condition known as hepatic encephalopathy), in the case of liver cirrhosis.

Probiotic supplements come in different forms—some need to be kept in the refrigerator; others don't—so choose the one that suits your lifestyle and follow the guidelines for storage. You'll want to buy supplements that contain multiple strains of beneficial bacteria, but first have a discussion with your doctor or dietitian about the strains that are best for the health condition you're treating; after all, different strains address different medical problems. If you're not ready to go the supplemental route, you can increase your intake of probiotic-rich dairy products by choosing those with live and active cultures, as well as consuming fermented foods, such as miso, tempeh, sauerkraut, and kombucha.

chapter 8

Reclaiming the Kitchen (and Your Eating Habits)

O N A BASIC, UTILITARIAN LEVEL, food serves as a source of sustenance and nourishment, as fuel for the cells in our organs (including the liver) and the energy we need to conduct our everyday life. But it's so much more than that. It's also a source of pleasure, comfort, and distraction, as well as a way to celebrate good news, express love, and show other people that we care. It's a form of social currency and cultural identity and so much more. Indeed, we live in a food-centric society, where eating and drinking are now incorporated into just about every social occasion imaginable. Given these realities, it's no wonder why it has become so challenging for many people to upgrade their eating habits. After all, no one likes to feel deprived of the foods he or she loves or feel left out of celebratory or social events.

The good news is you don't have to. It is possible to consume a healthy diet with many of your favorite foods—and still protect your liver, your weight, and your overall health. It isn't as difficult as it may sound at first, but it does require some planning and forethought. Both eating plans in Chapters 9 and 10 adhere to the principles described in Chapter 7, following a largely Mediterranean diet-style eating pattern, with lots of antioxidant-rich fruits and vegetables, fish and other foods that are loaded with omega-3 fatty acids, probiotics in fermented foods, and so on. But they also contain a little bit of everything to keep your taste buds pleased and your health well supported.

Because both plans are designed to protect the liver, they call for specific modifications to your diet that you might not expect. These include the following:

1. **Eliminate most white foods.** Tofu, cauliflower, onions, white beans, and hearts of palm can stay. But white bread, pasta, rice, and crackers, as well as white potatoes and other starchy or sugary foods, need to go because they cause your insulin and blood sugar to embark on a major roller-coaster ride, which over time increases your chances of developing insulin resistance and suffering liver damage. Note: Bean-based pastas, such as those made from black beans, red lentils, and edamame, are hot, as in trendy, right now; because they're loaded with protein (about 20 grams per serving) and fiber (usually more than 10 grams per serving) and have less carbs than traditional pasta, they won't take your insulin or blood sugar levels on a wild ride.

2. **Breakfast is not an option.** It's a requirement. I recommend starting the day with a protein source, such as eggs, and a vegetable several days a week, because the protein helps prevent cravings later and having a veggie helps set the tone of healthy eating for the day (plus, it gives you a leg up on your daily produce intake). On other days, start with a healthy source of whole grains or probiotics to fuel your body. Add coffee or green tea, and you've got an energizing morning meal!

3. **View trans fats as poisons.** They are essentially toxins because they're harmful to your blood vessels and damaging to your liver. Get in the habit of reading labels on packaged foods and avoid anything that has the words "partially hydrogenated oils" on it. Also, steer clear of fried foods, which often rely on hydrogenated oils to make French fries, onion rings, mozzarella sticks, and other fried fare.

4. **Upgrade your macronutrients.** Trade in simple carbs for complex ones (such as whole grains and veggies), high-fat sources of protein for lean ones (fish, tofu, eggs, legumes, and skinless poultry), and unhealthy fats for healthy monounsaturated and polyunsaturated ones (such as organic, cold-pressed olive oil, avocados, nuts, and seeds). While healthy carbs, protein, and fats will make your liver happy, starchy carbs, fat-filled protein, trans fats, and saturated fats will make it downright angry (and perhaps inflamed!).

5. **Include five different colored foods in your daily diet.** Brightly colored fruits and vegetables are loaded with antioxidants and

health-promoting plant compounds called phytochemicals. Foods with different hues (blueberries, oranges, red tomatoes, yellow bell peppers, spinach, purple eggplant, and so on) typically contain different types of phytochemicals. The more colors of produce there are in your diet, the merrier your health will be. So, choose a sweet potato instead of a white potato, and kale or even Romaine over iceberg lettuce.

6. **Eat till you're no longer hungry.** Contrary to what many people believe, the goal really isn't to become full (that's a sign that you've eaten too much). The goal is to be satisfied, as in pleasantly sated. A concept in the Okinawan culture, where people often live to be one hundred, is known as *hara hachi bu*: it instructs people to eat until they're 80 percent full. If you haven't done so already, I suggest you try this approach by eating slowly and mindfully, chewing your food well, and paying attention to your body's signals. This will help you achieve satisfaction without consuming unnecessary food and calories (while also sparing you the task of having to count them).

7. **Choose foods with fewer than six ingredients.** This strategy will help you curb your intake of highly processed foods that have additives, preservatives, fillers, and other artificial ingredients. If an ingredients list contains items you can't pronounce or can't identify, think twice about buying it and putting it in your body. As a general rule, foods that have relatively short ingredients lists tend to be more wholesome and nutritious. Stick with these!

8. **Opt for organic foods whenever possible.** Yes, they're often more expensive but not always by much, and often they're worth the added cost. After all, you'll be doing your body, especially your liver, a favor if you minimize your intake of pesticides. One of the best ways to do this is to rely on the Environmental Working Group's testing data for pesticide residue. Among the ten worst offenders: apples, peaches, nectarines, strawberries, grapes, celery, spinach, sweet bell peppers, cucumbers, and cherry tomatoes; these items are worth splurging on with the organic variety. Among the cleanest forms of produce: avocados, sweet corn, pineapple, cabbage, frozen sweet peas, onions, asparagus, mangoes, papayas, and kiwis—so, if you're looking to save a bit, these conventionally grown items are okay to buy. (Check out http://www.ewg.org for more information.)

As you saw in Chapter 4, certain foods wreak havoc on your liver by promoting internal inflammation, increasing fat storage, and contributing to further liver damage, such as fibrosis (scarring) and cirrhosis. Here are five foods to put on your no-fly list while you're trying to lose weight or just to improve your health.

Sugars or syrups Sugar, honey, cane juice, fruit juice concentrate, syrup of any kind, or anything ending in –ose are all forms of added sugar in packaged foods, such as crackers, condiments, soda, juice, granola bars, and cereals. When you eat them, they can cause massive spikes in blood sugar and insulin levels, which directly strain the liver. Fructose may be one of the worst offenders when it's added to foods, because processed fructose (such as high-fructose corn syrup and crystalline fructose) is directly converted to fat in the liver and may contribute to further inflammation and damage. (Don't worry about the fructose that comes from fresh fruits; because fruit contains fiber, the effects on blood sugar and insulin are not as extreme.)

Excess alcohol It's okay to have a glass of red wine once in a while. But too much alcohol puts a tremendous amount of stress on the liver. Most people realize that, but the threshold for how much is too much is probably lower than you think: "Excess" alcohol means more than one serving a day for women and more than two for men. If you already have nonalcoholic fatty liver disease (NAFLD) and are overweight, the added stress from alcohol could be too much for your liver to bear.

Trans fats Trans fats (in many packaged baked goods, creamed candies, and fried foods) have never been found to have a redeeming value, nutritionally speaking. What's worse, a 2010 study from the University of Cincinnati College of Medicine suggests that consuming trans fats in the diet can lead to fibrosis.

High sodium In people with existing liver damage—due to fatty liver disease or hepatitis, for instance—consuming excessive amounts of sodium may cause further damage to the liver. Since most of the sodium in our diets comes from processed foods (think: canned soup, salad dressings, and salty snacks such as chips and pretzels), sticking to a diet that relies on whole foods (such as the eating plans in Chapters 9 and 10 do), rather than packaged foods, will help you decrease your sodium intake significantly. It may seem hard to cut down on salt, but if you rely more on herbs and spices, your food will taste better and you'll find that you won't miss the salt.

White grains Any grain that has had its fiber removed is essentially devoid of nutrients and will elicit a response that's similar to the body's reaction to simple sugars: Dramatic spikes in blood sugar and insulin levels, which directly strain the liver, followed by rapid declines—a roller-coaster ride, in other words. Steer clear of white rice, breads, and pastas.

9. Get busy in the kitchen. Adopt the maxim "Cook more, dine out less," and you'll be better able to control your ingredients and your portions. When you eat out, it's easy to consume massive amounts of calories, carbs, and fats—an overload that's hard on your liver, your weight, and the rest of your body. Plan to eat at home at least six nights a week. Besides allowing you to prepare healthy meals, cooking allows you to add liver-friendly herbs and spices, such as turmeric (found in curry powder), cinnamon, and ginger, ingredients often included in the recipes that follow. In working with patients and clients, I have found that people are more likely to stick to a healthy eating regimen if they use herbs, spices, and roots that *they* love. While I've made suggestions on how to spice up your dishes in the meal ideas that follow, feel free to add seasonings that suit your taste buds—all herbs and spices have health benefits, so you really can't go wrong!

10. Embrace water as your new best friend. Consuming more water means you'll consume less soda, juice, or specialty drinks—a welcome improvement for your wallet and your calorie budget. My personal policy is to avoid drinking calories as much as possible because your body won't compensate for liquid calories by consuming fewer calories from food. Fluid calories can quickly add up to excess calories, contributing to weight gain. Plus, water helps keep the entire body functioning optimally, helping to regulate fluid and electrolyte balances, promoting good digestion, and more.

In Appendix C, you'll find a Healthy Liver Weekly Journal to help you monitor the changes you're making, challenges you're encountering, and how you could handle them differently.

Smart Swaps

To keep your liver (and the rest of your body) in top working order, you'll want to make some easy substitutions in your diet. Try making swaps gradually; you'll find yourself becoming more and more accustomed to liver-friendly foods—and you'll also find that many of them really taste better.

Here's a look at good ones to include:

Instead of:	Have:
White rice	Brown rice
Refined white or wheat bread	100% whole wheat or whole-grain bread
Instant oatmeal	Steel-cut oats
White or wheat pasta	100% whole-grain or bean-based pasta
Flour tortilla	Corn, almond, or brown rice tortilla
Refined white or wheat crackers	Grain-free, seed-based crackers
Plain bagel	Whole-grain English muffin
Raisins	Dried apricots
100% fruit juice	Whole fruit
White or baking potatoes	Sweet potatoes or yams
Iceberg lettuce	Dark leafy greens (spinach, kale, chard, mesclun, mustard greens)
Vegetable oil	Extra-virgin olive oil or organic, expeller-pressed canola oil
Red meat with a high fat content	Lean meats or fish
Chicken thigh (dark meat)	Chicken breast (white meat)
Chocolate-covered nuts and seeds	Raw nuts and seeds
Honey-roasted nuts	Unsweetened cinnamon or cocoa nuts
Hamburgers	Homemade black bean burgers
Farmed seafood	Wild-caught seafood
Yogurt sweetened with sugar or sucralose	Full-fat or low-fat yogurt, unsweetened or sweetened with stevia
Kefir sweetened with sugar or sucralose	Unsweetened kefir
Processed cheeses	Aged cheeses, such as Parmesan
Cappuccino or mocha drinks	Black coffee (may add unsweetened almond milk and stevia)
Chai tea latte	Hot green tea
Pop or soda	Unsweetened carbonated beverages with natural flavoring
Sweet tea	Unsweetened iced tea with lemon
Sugary or sweetened cocktails	Red wine
Bottled salad dressings	Good-quality olive oil and balsamic vinegar
Sweet teriyaki sauce	Reduced-sodium soy sauce
Ketchup	Yellow or Dijon mustard
Mayonnaise	Avocado or hummus spread
Cream-based sauce or dressing	Tahini
Flavor packets	Lemon or lime juice
Milk chocolate	Dark chocolate (>72% cacao)
Milk shake	Blended milk, ripe banana, and cacao
Regular or tapioca pudding	Homemade chia pudding
Slice of fruit pie	Berries with melted dark chocolate
Products sweetened with sucralose	Products sweetened with stevia
Pasta noodles	Spaghetti squash or spiralized veggies
All fruit smoothie	Green smoothie with protein
Pancakes with syrup	Whole-grain French toast with berries

Smart Kitchen Makeover Strategies

For many people, the kitchen is the hub of their home, the main gathering place and the setting where you're most likely to eat and socialize. To feed your liver the foods that will help it thrive, you'll want to set up your kitchen in a way that encourages healthy eating—by keeping the good stuff readily available—and discourages the consumption of foods that aren't good for your liver. That's where the concept of giving your kitchen a makeover comes in. You won't need a contractor or a carpenter for this version, just a methodical, organized approach to structuring your kitchen so it supports your liver-protection goals.

To that end, it's wise to keep your kitchen counters clear of temptations and junk foods that may trigger the urge to nosh when you're not particularly hungry. So, put the cookie jar behind closed (cabinet) doors! If you want to keep anything in plain sight, stick with brightly colored fruits in a bowl. A 2012 study from St. Bonaventure University in New York found that when fruits are placed in a visible bowl in the kitchen, residents increased their consumption of these nutrient-rich foods.

In the fall of 2015, a young man named AJ, 20, was sent to me by his mother. AJ was morbidly obese. He was gearing up to go back to college and was preparing to move into an apartment on campus, where he'd have the opportunity to buy and cook his own food—and hopefully lose some of the weight he'd put on the previous year while eating in the food hall. One of the first things we did was help him learn how to stock his kitchen healthfully, with basic pantry items and freezer staples he could keep on hand to make quick, healthy meals in a pinch (thus avoiding a call to the pizza delivery man). Then, we went to the grocery store where we focused on shopping the perimeter, picking good sources of lean protein (such as wild fish and grass-fed beef) and produce, before traversing the aisles to find healthy fats, whole grains, and essential canned items. After our kitchen makeover and grocery store tour, AJ felt more confident than ever in setting up his environment for success.

When we met again a year later, AJ had lost 50 pounds simply by becoming a savvier shopper and changing the way he chose and prepared food. He also curtailed his drinking that year—and had a girlfriend who enjoyed cooking with him. College life had taken a turn for the better (and healthier)!

What follows are the best ways to organize two primary areas in your kitchen—the fridge and the pantry. Before you get started, buy sandwich bags and other portion-controlled containers so you can put certain foods in individual compartments; you'll need to be able to do this to fulfill some of the recommended tactics.

The Fridge

Rule number one: Make sure your refrigerator and freezer are at the proper temperatures to keep your perishable foods fresh. The fridge should be kept below 40°F, the freezer at 0°F. Don't just rely on the control setting; buy an inexpensive appliance thermometer so you can keep tabs on the temperatures. When you come home from the grocery store, store perishable items right away, and adhere to the "two-hour rule": Don't leave meat, poultry, seafood, eggs, dairy products, or other items that need refrigeration at room temperature for longer than two hours, a max of one hour in hot weather (these rules apply to leftovers and take-out fare, too).

Once this bit of housekeeping is taken care of, here are the best ways to set up your refrigerator:

Start cutting ahead of time One excuse I frequently hear from patients has to do with not having the time to prepare fresh produce so that it can be easily consumed. To make this a cinch, I recommend buying whole organic carrots or celery stalks, which need to be washed and peeled (in the case of carrots), and cutting them up in advance. You can keep them fresh by wrapping them in paper towels and placing them in breathable plastic bags for up to five days in your fridge. This will make it easy to grab them for a quick snack or it can give you a head start on meal preparation.

Use containers strategically Put healthy items in clear glass, and those unhealthy ones in opaque plastic or ceramic containers. This way, the healthy leftovers and prepared foods will be seen easily, while the less-than-healthy leftover cake or fried foods won't be. If you have the space, I suggest storing leftovers in preportioned, smaller containers so you can just grab them and heat them, instead of having to portion out a serving from a huge container when it's time to eat.

Keep protein accessible Have small portions of protein—such as sticks of string cheese, yogurt, peanut butter balls in single-serving resealable plastic bags (see page 257 for the recipe), hard-boiled eggs, and the like—within easy reach for a quick grab-and-go snack.

Place produce in plain sight Out of sight tends to mean out of mind, so rather than putting your produce in the drawers, store colorful fruits and vegetables on the shelves at eye level (perhaps near dips or spreads, such as low-fat yogurt, hummus, and guacamole). Instead, use the drawers for unhealthier items (such as leftover lasagna) or refrigerated desserts. Just as grocery stores use strategic placement of products to make you more likely to buy them, you can use the same principle with healthier items in your fridge.

Use the door of your fridge wisely Don't store eggs or dairy products on the door as these items are easily perishable. Instead, place liver-friendly condiments—such as hot sauce (which contains capsaicin), yellow mustard (which contains turmeric), horseradish, Asian fish sauce, and gluten-free soy sauce—on the door for easy access.

Stock your freezer It's the perfect place to store frozen fruits and vegetables that you can use at a moment's notice. It's also a place where things get "burned," an unfortunate state that's often discovered when you clean out your freezer. To prevent this, make sure you store your vegetables and lean meats up front and center so it's easy to remember that they're there. Always keep at least one frozen vegetable on hand (such as broccoli) that you can grab if your fridge runs out of fresh produce. If you often take your lunch to work, consider placing single-serving homemade foods (as in leftovers!) in containers that you can easily pack up.

TRY TO WASTE NOT . . . BUT KNOW WHEN TO TOSS IT!

When it comes to determining whether foods are truly past their prime, there's massive confusion among consumers. A 2011 survey by the Food Marketing Institute found that 91 percent of consumers said that they had thrown out food on its "sell by" date because they were concerned that it had become unsafe to eat. Well, here's a surprise: The dates on food product labels—including "sell by," "use by," and "best before" dates—don't necessarily mean what you think they do; they are merely suggestions from manufacturers about when a food item reaches peak quality, not an indication of whether it's safe to eat it (or not). Only an "expiration date" relates to food safety, so if an item has passed that date, throw it out.

Some general rules of thumb to keep in mind for perishable items that require refrigeration:

- Milk is usually safe to use for 2 to 3 days after the "use by" date; keep it in the back of the fridge where the temperature is coldest.
- Eggs can be safely consumed for several weeks after the "sell by" date on the carton.
- Unopened yogurt and cottage cheese can be consumed 14 days after the "best buy" or "sell by" date on the package.
- Raw fish, fresh (not frozen) poultry, and ground beef should be cooked and consumed within 2 days of purchase.
- Luncheon meats should be consumed within 3 to 5 days of opening the package; the same goes for freshly sliced meats from the deli.

If there's ever a question about whether a food item is fit for consumption, let your senses guide you: If it has turned a funky color or it has curdled, or if it smells rotten or rancid, your best bet is to toss it in the trash or compost it—without tasting it "to be sure."

The Pantry

For starters, it's best to adhere to a first-in, last-out approach. In food science class in nutrition school, we learned that the longest-lasting foods should be placed in the back of the pantry and the ones that are most likely to go bad or turn stale sooner should be in the front. To help guide your food choices, you can use this principle with healthy (lower calorie, lower sugar) items, as well. If you do, your cabinets or pantry might feature long containers that store your preportioned baggies of nuts and popcorn in front; at the back you'd find 1-ounce bars of dark chocolate. Both items are healthy but the popcorn and nuts are better as a readily available, satisfying grab-and-go snack, while the dark chocolate is best suited as a once-in-a-while treat, which is why you should have to look for it to get your hands on it.

Other smart ways to set up your pantry:

Minimize variety It may be the spice of life but when it comes to food, having too much variety can make you likely to eat more—and choose unhealthier items. So, curb your choices, particularly when it comes to crackers, snack foods, and cereals, and you'll improve your odds of sticking with your good-eating intentions.

Remember: Bulk items can create . . . bulk! Yes, buying in bulk can help you save money—but it can also make you eat in bulk. Which isn't what you want! The solution is to take an oversize bag of popcorn or a huge box of cereal, and divide the contents into individual portions in small bags. If you want to motivate yourself further, you might write something on the bag in permanent marker—such as "savor the flavor" or "chew slowly"—that will help you stay accountable with your planned intake.

Stock up on staples To keep a ready supply of healthy ingredients handy so you can assemble delicious, nutritious meals in a flash, fill your pantry with the following essentials:

- Canned or Tetra Pak goods: No-added-sugar tomato sauce, diced tomatoes, crushed tomatoes, tomato paste, tomato puree, pumpkin, canned wild salmon, canned sardines, canned tuna; low-sodium black beans, pinto beans, red beans, garbanzo beans (chickpeas), lentils, fat-free refried beans, organic coconut milk, low-sodium broth-based soups. Since the lining of many cans contains BPA, you can also look for these goods packaged in Tetra Paks.

THE CALORIE CONUNDRUM

You've probably heard the expression that "a calorie is a calorie," and it's true that any calorie that's left over after we've used the calories we need for energy will be stored as fat. But that's as far as the validity of the equality argument goes. The reality is while all calories give us energy, not all calories are created equal, and certain organs, including your liver, are especially picky about the calories you consume. As far as your liver and heart are concerned, calories from fiber-rich foods (such as whole grains, legumes, veggies, and fruits), antioxidant-packed foods (such as colorful fruits and veggies), lean protein sources (such as fish, seafood, skinless chicken or turkey breast, eggs, legumes, nuts, seeds, and low-fat dairy products), and healthy fats (as in monounsaturated and polyunsaturated fats) trump all others. These calories should dominate your diet 90 percent of the time; the other 10 percent can be considered "discretionary" calories, from treats or occasional indulgences (such as a scoop of ice cream or a slice of birthday cake).

The journey to improved health and a trimmer waistline starts with eating the right foods (ones that are health-promoting) and avoiding the wrong foods (ones that can hijack your appetite, your weight, and your health). The eating plans outlined in this book don't focus on the number of calories, but instead on the nutrient density of your calories. This is because healthy sources of calories will fill you up and make you less likely to overeat. So, let nourishing foods take center stage in your life and pay attention to the effects these nutritional all-stars have on your body, including how you feel and function, and over time you'll feel less tempted by junk food and other unhealthy fare. Feeling good really can be self-reinforcing and practically addictive!

- Pastas: Bean-based pastas (such as black bean, red lentil, and edamame), brown rice pasta, 100% whole wheat pasta
- Rice and whole grains: Brown rice, red rice, black rice, wild rice, freekeh, farro, barley, whole wheat pearled couscous, millet
- Healthy snacks: Flaxseed crackers, spelt pretzels, raw unsweetened coconut chips, bags of prepopped popcorn (with just oil or salt or air-popped)
- Nondairy milks (that don't need to be refrigerated until opened): Unsweetened almond milk, unsweetened cashew milk, unsweetened hemp milk

- Oils and fats: Olive oil, coconut oil, avocado oil
- Vinegars: Balsamic vinegar, cider vinegar, white wine vinegar, rice vinegar
- Herbs and spices: Oregano, rosemary, turmeric, or curry powder, black pepper, thyme, cinnamon, cumin, chili powder, paprika
- Nuts and seeds: Unsalted raw almonds, unsalted peanuts, no-added-sugar peanut butter, almond butter, cashew butter, unsalted raw cashews, unsalted pistachios, chia seeds, flaxseeds
- Miscellaneous: Vegan protein powder, whey protein powder, dried peas and beans

From freekeh to miso: some new ingredients Some of the foods in the meal plans that follow may be new to you (and your liver). Most of them can be found in your usual grocery store or your local Whole Foods Market or natural food store. All of them can be found online (often in bulk and less expensively). Here's a short guide to what these unusual foods are and how to use them.

Almond flour Almond flour is a gluten-free flour made from turning almonds into meal by blanching the almonds to remove the skin then grinding them into a fine texture. Almond flour is higher in fat than regular all-purpose flour yet lower in carbohydrates; in addition, it boasts a high amount of vitamin E and on average about 6 grams of protein per serving. You can buy almond flour at any grocery store, but better yet, you can make almond flour in your own kitchen with raw almonds and a good-quality blender.

Almond protein crackers Instead of using grains, these crackers are made from almonds (and other nuts) as well as seeds and spices to create a crunchy, flavorful snack that packs a lot of protein. Many grocery stores carry these crackers; they are often stocked near the gluten-free products.

Ancient grains Such grains as quinoa, spelt, millet, barley, bulgur, freekeh, farro, kamut, amaranth, and buckwheat are considered "ancient" because little about them has changed over the thousands of years since humans began consuming them. This is in contrast to more commercial crops, such as wheat and corn, which have been altered dramatically from their original forms due to selective breeding in agriculture. Ancient grains are excellent sources of whole intact grain and fiber and are often higher in protein and micronutrients as well. Most of these are as easy to prepare as white rice—and make a great swap to add more nutrition—and taste—to your meals.

Bean-based pasta Now available in many traditional grocery stores, these pasta-shaped noodles are made entirely of black beans, soybeans, lentils, or other legumes. Bean-based pastas add both protein and fiber and decrease carbs in a meal as well. They can be used similarly to traditional pastas, but the texture may vary depending on the type of bean used. They are entirely grain-free!

Black rice Sometimes called forbidden rice, black rice has a nutty, earthy taste. It's loaded with fiber and B vitamins, and research suggests it may contain more cancer-fighting antioxidants than blueberries or blackberries do. You can find black rice in most health-food stores and you can use it in place of other types of rice in recipes.

Broccolini A hybrid between regular broccoli and Chinese broccoli (*gai-lan*), broccolini has smaller florets and longer, thinner stalks and a slightly sweeter flavor and more tender texture than broccoli. It has a similar nutritional profile to broccoli and can be sautéed, steamed, roasted, or grilled. You'll find it in the produce section.

Brown rice tortillas Made using brown rice instead of wheat flour or corn, brown rice tortillas offer an alternative source of whole grains and a lot of fiber while maintaining the same functionality as traditional tortillas. They can be found in the breads area of many health-food stores and with gluten-free products in traditional grocery stores.

Cacao powder A powder made from grinding up whole, roasted cacao beans that are used to make chocolate, cacao powder can provide the flavor of chocolate in shakes and smoothies—without the additives contained in commercial chocolate. With a flavor that's richer and bitterer than milk chocolate, cacao powder is a good source of potassium, zinc, and antioxidants. Health-food stores carry cacao powder in packets or bags.

Chia seeds An ancient Mexican seed from the *Salvia hispanica* plant, chia seeds provide a plant-based source of omega-3 fatty acids (in addition to fiber and protein) that works well in smoothies, salads, and rice dishes. It also can be used to thicken soups and sauces, since it swells into a gel-like substance when it's submerged in liquid. Unlike flaxseeds, chia seeds do not need to be ground first to obtain the omega-3 benefits. Chia seeds can be found in most grocery stores these days.

Coconut shreds Also called desiccated coconut, these are dried shreds that can be easily added to smoothies and salads or used in baking. Coconut shreds are sold by the bag in most grocery stores as well as in bulk in health-food stores; before purchasing, check the ingredients and choose a brand that does not have added sugar.

Edamame A fancy name for young soybeans that have been harvested before the beans have had a chance to harden, edamame are usually boiled or steamed in the pod and served with salt. Often used in Japanese cuisine, edamame have become fairly popular as a side dish or snack in the United States, too. They are a great addition to salads (you can even make an edamame-based dip). You'll find them fresh or frozen in most grocery stores.

Hemp hearts These are the inner portion of hemp seeds, or "hulled" hemp seeds, which are more easily digested. Hemp hearts, which have a rich, nutty flavor similar to pine nuts, are an excellent source of plant-based omega-3 and omega-6 fatty acids and they are a complete protein. They can be tossed into salads, protein shakes, oatmeal, or many other meals for a nutritional boost.

Infused olive oil A variety of extra-virgin olive oils are available, including some that are infused with added flavors, such as basil, lemon, garlic, or rosemary. Because these olive oils provide flavor without additional ingredients or calories, they're a great option for homemade salad dressings.

Jicama A root vegetable that looks like a cross between a potato and a turnip, raw jicama has a slightly sweet flavor and a crunchy texture that's similar to a water chestnut. High in vitamin C and fiber, it's very low in fat and when shredded or sliced thinly, a great addition to salads or wraps. You'll find jicama in the produce section of most grocery stores.

Kefir A fermented milk-based product, kefir is a great source of probiotics and protein. It has a similar flavor to yogurt but a much thinner, beverage-like consistency. It can be consumed plain, used in recipes, or blended into smoothies. Kefir is available in most grocery stores, typically in quart-size bottles in the dairy section. Dairy-free kefir is also available.

Leeks Along with chives, garlic, onions, and shallots, leeks are members of the Allium vegetable family (they look like extra-large scallions). Slicing and sautéing or grilling them really brings out their sweet, fragrant flavor. They can be eaten on their own or added to many different dishes. You'll find them in the produce section of most grocery stores.

Milk alternatives For those who can't (or don't want to) drink cow's milk, a variety of nondairy alternatives are widely available—and they're growing in popularity due to their high nutrient content; plus, they often have fewer calories and less sugar (as long as you choose the unsweetened ones). In particular, unsweetened vanilla almond milk is a delicious option, with only 30 calories per cup and a creamy texture. Others include soy milk, coconut milk, cashew milk, and rice milk. Many of these come in shelf-stable cartons that don't need to be refrigerated until they're opened.

Miso A salty paste that's derived from fermented soybeans, salt, and rice malt, miso comes in red, brown, yellow, or white varieties. It's commonly used to make miso soup, but it also can be added to salad dressings, mixed with avocado for a condiment, and even added to stews and other soups. It's a great source of isoflavones, B vitamins, probiotics, and enzymes.

Nutritional yeast Typically used as an alternative to cheese in vegan diets, nutritional yeast is a deactivated yeast that comes in flakes and is sold in health-food stores. It does not leaven breads and other baked goods as activated yeast does; instead, it can be used as a topping in place of Parmesan cheese. It has a cheesy, nutty flavor.

Protein powders Offering an easy way to increase your protein intake without adding lots of fat, protein powders, which range from plant-based sources (such as soy and pea) to dairy and egg sources (such as whey and egg white), are typically added to smoothies but also can be used in yogurt parfaits or homemade energy bars. When shopping for a protein powder, look for those with the shortest ingredients lists and avoid ingredients you can't pronounce, as well as those with artificial flavors, sweeteners, and colors or a long list of herbs and supplements. Protein powders are typically sold in health-food stores or mega-department stores (such as Target or Walmart).

Quinoa A whole grain that can be used in a similar fashion to rice since it has a mild flavor, quinoa is the only grain that is a complete protein. In recent years, it has grown in popularity in the United States and is widely available in grocery stores.

Sea vegetables Algae, nori and other seaweed, and spirulina are highly nutritious and can be easily added to protein shakes, salads, stir-fries, and other recipes. Dehydrated seaweed is sold in packets of varying sizes in most grocery stores (look in the international and ethnic food aisle). Different types have different flavors, but most are fairly mild, which means you can use them similarly to other greens. In the recipes that follow, you'll find sea vegetables listed as "sea-weed," "nori," or "spirulina."

"Spiralized" vegetables An inexpensive device that can be pur-chased at home goods stores or online, a spiralizer can transform fresh veggies—such as zucchini, carrots, and cucumbers—into long, thin strands that look like noodles. Spiralized vegetables have a great texture, especially when they're substituted for pasta.

Sprouted seeds Seeds that have started to germinate or "sprout," sprouted seeds pack a lot of nutrients in a small package. Chances are, you're familiar with alfalfa sprouts or sprouted soybeans (a.k.a. bean sprouts); many other beans and seeds—including lentils, peas, chickpeas, and sunflower seeds—can be prepared this way. In addi-tion, some whole-grain breads contain sprouted seeds. Sprouts are a great addition to salads and sandwiches.

Tahini A paste made from sesame seeds, tahini has lots of copper and magnesium, both of which are needed to keep the body in tip-top shape, as well as high amounts of calcium and zinc. While you might be familiar with tahini as an ingredient in hummus, it's also an amazing addition to sauces, dressings, stews, soups, marinades, and even baked goods. You can find it in most grocery stores.

Tempeh A plant-based protein source that's made from soy-beans, tempeh is stiffer than tofu and it has a nutty flavor. It is also a fermented food and therefore a great dietary source of probiotics. You'll find it in the (refrigerated) vegetarian section of most grocery stores.

Wasabi powder A staple in sushi, wasabi is a type of Japanese horseradish with a strong, spicy taste. When it's dried, it's made into a powder that can easily be added to dressings, marinades, and sauces. It can be found in specialty spice stores, Asian markets, and some health-food stores.

Za'atar This tasty Middle Eastern mixture of sumac seeds, thyme, salt, and sesame seeds can be sprinkled on flatbread, eggs, or steamed vegetables; mixed into a marinade for chicken; or sprinkled into extra-virgin olive oil and used as a dip for whole-grain bread. Besides offering a delicious flavor infusion, sumac berries and thyme have been linked to a decreased incidence of foodborne pathogens. Za'atar can be found in spice stores, Middle Eastern markets, and many grocery stores in the spice aisle.

Taking Your Healthy Diet on the Road

While setting up a healthy home is essential for a healthy liver, we can't stay home every day in our comfortable, well-controlled environment. We have jobs, travel plans, social obligations, and schedules that take us out of our environment and throw us into others. To stay on track with your liver-protection plan, you'll need to arm yourself with tools and tactics to help you survive in the outside world. To help you (and your liver) stay in better shape when you're relying on someone else to cook your food, take the following steps:

Plan ahead Many restaurants now post their menus and nutritional information online, giving you the opportunity to choose both a restaurant and a meal that will fit into your healthy eating plan. Choose establishments with varied menus and avoid all-you-can-eat buffets or places where fried foods dominate more than half the menu. Once you've chosen a restaurant, call ahead and ask such questions as: "Is the chef able to alter menu items based on specific dietary needs or requests?" or "Can I bring my own salad dressing?"

Make reservations when you can If you arrive at a restaurant and discover that there's an hour's wait for a table, you're likely to become extremely hungry even if you had a snack ahead of time. Or, you may head to the bar to grab a drink and maybe have an appetizer while you wait. You may even change your ordering plan when you see and smell what other diners are having. The upshot: All your good planning flies out the window, all because you weren't able to sit down immediately. Having a reservation can prevent this scenario from occurring. (It's a good idea to bring along a small snack—such as a single-serving-size bag of almonds—just in case.)

Snack first When you show up at a restaurant feeling ravenous, it's easy to overeat (especially if you don't have a reservation and have to wait for a table!). That's why it's smart to have a small snack ahead of time. Eating one that includes a protein and a complex carbohydrate (such as low-fat yogurt and berries or hummus and baby carrots) beforehand should help you walk into a restaurant with your restraint intact.

Establish an "at the table" model for success For starters, be the first person at the table to order because peer pressure doesn't end in high school. Research suggests that if you're with a group of people, ordering first can help you stay true to what you want to eat and avoid being influenced by what someone else orders. To reduce portions, it helps to find an ally with whom you can split an entrée. Don't hesitate to create your own meal: People often consider "sides" as ways to enhance their main course, but you can put together a healthy, plant-based meal by combining a couple of side dishes that appeal to you, in place of ordering an entrée.

Question your server (but don't be a jerk) Don't be shy about asking questions to determine what's really in a particular dish. If something is served with a "light sauce," don't take the description at face value: ask what's in it. Also, don't be afraid to make special requests, such as asking that a piece of fish be broiled or grilled instead of fried, to have a pasta dish with extra veggies and less pasta, or to ask to have a sauce on the side rather than on the fish or that something be prepared with olive oil instead of butter.

Eat and drink slowly Maintain the mindful eating practices you've been using at home by slowing down your eating, putting your fork down between bites, and enjoying the other important aspects of the meal—such as the conversation and company of your companions. If you drink alcohol, limit yourself to one cocktail or glass of wine or beer and allow plenty of sips of water between each sip of alcohol.

Be choosy about desserts If you're asked if you'd like to see a dessert menu, politely decline the offer, saying you're too full after the delicious meal. If you must have dessert, choose fresh fruit (such as mixed berries) or sorbet. Or split a richer dessert with one of your dining companions and enjoy a few bites. We all deserve an indulgence once in a while; the key is to limit the quantity you consume.

By giving your kitchen a makeover, regularly incorporating these tasty, good-for-you foods into your meals, and dining smartly at restaurants, you'll be providing your body with the right fuel so you can feel and function at your best. Whether you want to improve your diet to lose weight or simply to protect your liver (along with the rest of your body), you'll want to put the principles you've just read about into practice. In the next two chapters, you'll get the inside scoop on how to make these strategies work for your personal goals.

part three

Creating a Healthy Future for Your Liver

chapter 9

The Love-Your-Liver Eating Plan

W HEN IT COMES TO improving their eating habits, many people think this means they'll feel perpetually hungry or they'll have to deprive themselves of tasty foods. That's just not true! As you saw in the previous chapters, it is entirely possible to stick with a healthy eating regimen that provides lots of nutrients and plenty of pleasure while protecting your liver, your overall health, and your weight. As you've learned, as far as your liver is concerned the key to eating right is to consume lots of nutrient-packed, antioxidant-rich foods that support your liver and avoid foods that could harm this vital organ.

The four-week plan that follows is designed to help you maintain your weight, whereas the plan in Chapter 10 is formulated to help you lose weight. Even though calorie-counting isn't part of the equation, in case you're curious, this one contains roughly 1,800 to 2,100 calories per day: 400 to 500 each for breakfast, lunch, and dinner, plus 400 to 500 for snacks and treats. You should choose this plan if your weight is in the normal range (or close to it)—whether it's always been there or you've lost weight and now want to maintain your current weight—and want to enhance the health of your liver.

The following meal plans and recipes will provide you with your fill of health-promoting foods. They're delicious, easy to prepare, and satisfying. By eliminating foods that are likely to offend your liver and feeding this precious organ foods that will help it thrive, you'll be boosting the powers of the magician behind the curtain, the one that controls much of the fate of your health, in incredible ways. The four-week plan lists more than eighty meals and snacks to choose from. These menu offerings will give you a powerful nutritional bang for every bite. (Your taste buds will be pretty darn satisfied, too!)

A few quick notes about drinks and snacks:

Drinks Have lots of water and calorie-free beverages (such as seltzer with a wedge of lemon or lime or iced tea), as well as hot tea and coffee if you enjoy these beverages.

Snacks Need a snack? Stick with the liver-loving foods you've learned about already, such as nuts, fruits, hummus, or even a small piece of dark chocolate.

If you want to lose weight, your best bet is to turn to the diet plan in Chapter 10. Bon appétit!

Note: You'll find that all the recipes in the plan below with an * are marked **LYL** in Appendix A, Recipes, at the back of the book.

WEEK 1

Sunday

BREAKFAST: 2 slices cinnamon-blackberry French toast (made with whole-grain bread dipped in 2 eggs, mixed with ground cinnamon and 2 tablespoons low-fat yogurt and cooked in 2 teaspoons coconut oil, then topped with ½ cup fresh blackberries)

LUNCH: Peanut butter and fruit roll (made by smearing 2 tablespoons no-added-sugar peanut butter on a whole-grain wrap and topping it with ½ cup strawberry or banana slices); on the side, ½ cup apple slices with ground cinnamon *or* a 6-ounce plain yogurt

DINNER: 1 cup Chicken Stir-fry with Asparagus, Peppers, and Cashews* over 1 cup cooked freekeh or quinoa

SNACK: ½ banana, sliced, with 1 ounce melted dark chocolate drizzled on top *or* ½ cup watermelon

Monday

BREAKFAST: 1 cup steel-cut oatmeal, cooked in unsweetened almond or cashew milk with ground cinnamon, a handful of walnuts, and ½ sliced banana

LUNCH: 1 serving Green Bean and Quinoa Bowl*

DINNER: 4 ounces poached salmon with ½ Baked Artichoke* and ½ cup wild rice pilaf

SNACK: 1 medium-size apple with 1 tablespoon no-added-sugar peanut butter or 3 whole carrots, cut into sticks, with ½ cup White Bean Hummus*

Tuesday
BREAKFAST: An 8-ounce kefir smoothie (place ½ cup kefir, ½ cup blueberries and/or raspberries, and 1 teaspoon honey in a blender and mix to desired consistency; 1 teaspoon whey protein powder, optional)

LUNCH: 2 cups seared bok choy, mixed with ½ cup Garlicky Tofu* and 1 cup cooked brown rice

DINNER: 1 cup whole wheat spaghetti, topped with 3 Spinach Turkey Meatballs*, 1 cup wilted kale, and 1 cup no-added-sugar tomato sauce, side of steamed broccoli

DESSERT OR TREAT: 1 Avocado Brownie Bite*

SNACK: 1 ounce soy nuts *or* 1 cup low-fat yogurt topped with ½ cup raspberries and 1 tablespoon chia seeds

Wednesday
BREAKFAST: Breakfast burrito, made with 1 egg scrambled in 1 tablespoon olive oil, mixed with ½ cup chopped tomato, 2 tablespoons parsley, and ¼ cup black beans and wrapped in a whole wheat or brown rice tortilla

LUNCH: 1 cup Mango, Avocado, and Black Bean Salad* with 1 tablespoon hemp hearts

DINNER: 1 cup Easy Corn Soup*, 4 ounces tuna seared in 1 tablespoon olive oil with Dandelion Greens Salad*

SNACK: 8-ounce Green Smoothie* *or* 10 to 12 whole-grain crackers with 1 tablespoon almond butter

Thursday
BREAKFAST: Yogurt parfait made with 1 cup low-fat yogurt, ¼ cup blueberries, ¼ cup raspberries, ¼ cup blackberries, and 1 ounce chopped walnuts

LUNCH: 4 ounces grilled chicken with 1 cup braised broccoli over 1 cup cooked quinoa

DINNER: 2 Fish Tacos*, plus ½ cup baked tortilla chips, ½ cup salsa, and ¼ cup guacamole on the side

SNACK: Green tea and a medium-size orange *or* apple

Friday

BREAKFAST: Florentine egg sandwich made with 1 egg fried in 1 teaspoon olive oil, with ¼ cup spinach on a 100% whole wheat roll

LUNCH: Tempeh sandwich (a 4-ounce piece of tempeh, any flavor, seared in 1 tablespoon olive oil, 2 slices 100% whole-grain sourdough bread) with 1 cup Roasted Brussels Sprouts* with garlic

DINNER: 1 Chia Lentil Burger*, topped with ½ cup spinach, 1 tomato slice, and 2 tablespoons chopped basil on a whole-grain bun, 1 cup baked sweet potato fries

SNACK: ½ cup homemade Roasted Beet Chips* *or* 1 ounce raw almonds

Saturday

BREAKFAST: Scrambled eggs (1 egg plus 2 egg whites) on top of 4 ounces smoked salmon; ½ cup fresh strawberries on the side

LUNCH: 1 cup cooked quinoa, made with unsweetened almond milk, with chopped apples, ¼ teaspoon ground cinnamon, and 1 ounce chopped pecans

DINNER: Pita pizza with vegetables (2 whole wheat pita halves, each with ¼ cup low- sugar pizza sauce, 2 tablespoons mozzarella cheese, and 3 leaves of spinach, cooked in toaster oven), 2 cups salad greens with 2 tablespoons balsamic dressing

SNACK: ¼ cup Edamame Hummus* with 10 to 12 whole-grain crackers *or* 1 medium-size Zucchini Muffin*

WEEK 2

Sunday

BREAKFAST: 1 soft-boiled egg with ½ avocado, sliced, and a 100% whole wheat English muffin (add 1 tablespoon olive oil to toasted muffin)

LUNCH: 1 cup steel-cut oats, cooked in unsweetened almond milk with a handful of slivered almonds and ½ cup chopped apple

DINNER: 2 cups spiralized zucchini with 1 cup no-added-sugar tomato sauce, 2 tablespoons Parmesan cheese, and 4 ounces grilled chicken or wild salmon

SNACK: 6 dark chocolate-covered apricots *or* a whole banana with 1 tablespoon no-added-sugar peanut butter

Monday

BREAKFAST: 1 cup shredded wheat cereal with 2 tablespoons chopped walnuts, ½ cup blueberries, and 1 cup unsweetened almond milk

LUNCH: Wild salmon patty (grilled or panfried) on a whole wheat bun with a side of arugula and tomatoes (1 cup arugula, ½ cup whole cherry tomatoes, and 2 tablespoons lemon-infused olive oil)

DINNER: 4 ounce grilled chicken breast with 1 cup beet and orange salad over cooked quinoa

SNACK: 15 grain-free almond protein crackers with ½ cup low-fat cottage cheese *or* 1 cup low-fat plain Greek yogurt with ½ cup raspberries and 1 tablespoon honey or a handful of walnuts

Tuesday

BREAKFAST: 1 cup Overnight-Soaked Oats* with almond butter

LUNCH: Tempeh sandwich (a 4-ounce piece of tempeh, any flavor, seared in 1 tablespoon olive oil, on 2 slices 100% whole-grain sourdough bread with 2 tablespoons Avocado Smear* and ½ cup spinach on top)

DINNER: 1 cup cooked brown rice with 1 tablespoon garlic-infused olive oil with ½ cup red kidney beans mixed in (reserve about 1 tablespoon of the liquid from the bean can and mix into brown rice); heat the mixture in a pan and add 2 cups kale until wilted

SNACK: 2 Peanut Butter Balls* *or* 1 organic Honey Crisp apple with 2 tablespoons no-added-sugar peanut butter and ground cinnamon

Wednesday

BREAKFAST: Scrambled eggs (1 whole egg and 1 egg white) in 1 tablespoon coconut oil with 2 slices whole-grain toast and ½ cup strawberries

LUNCH: 1 cup Black Bean Soup* topped with 2 tablespoons low-fat plain Greek yogurt and chopped cilantro

DINNER: A 5-ounce piece of wild salmon, pan-seared, served with ½ cup edamame pasta with 2 tablespoons jarred pesto sauce and 1 cup steamed broccoli

SNACK: A 1-ounce square of 70% cacao dark chocolate with ½ cup blackberries or 3½ cups bagged popcorn (plain variety with simply oil and sea salt)

Thursday

BREAKFAST: 1 whole wheat English muffin with 2 tablespoons natural cashew butter and a side of ½ cup chopped apple

LUNCH: 2 cups mesclun salad mix or a spinach-and-kale mix with ½ avocado, chopped, ¼ cup chopped orange bell pepper, and 2 tablespoons sprouted pumpkin seeds with 2 ½ tablespoons olive oil and 1 tablespoon fig balsamic vinegar with a 4-ounce piece of grilled chicken, sliced

DINNER: Tofu bean tacos (use ½ cup black beans from the previous day's soup; add ½ cup cubed tofu sautéed in 1 tablespoon olive oil and place in 2 corn tortillas), garnished with low-fat Cheddar cheese, scallions, and chopped tomatoes on top

SNACKS: ¼ cup Hummus* with 15 grain-free seed crackers or 1 cup carrot sticks; or a stick of string cheese with 1 pear

Friday

BREAKFAST: Yogurt parfait (1 cup low-fat plain Greek yogurt with ½ cup mixed berries, 1 teaspoon pure maple syrup and 2 tablespoons slivered almonds)

LUNCH: Turkey and Swiss chard roll-ups (roll 4 ounces sliced nitrate-free turkey with Swiss chard strips, enough to cover, divvy up 1 slice organic white Cheddar cheese and 1½ tablespoons Avocado Smear*)

DINNER: 1 cup Lemony Soybean Spaghetti with Arugula,* topped with 2 tablespoons hemp seeds

SNACK: 1 cup low-fat cottage cheese with 1 tablespoon honey *or* ½ cup raspberries and 1 to 2 handfuls of raw almond slivers

Saturday

BREAKFAST: 2 small wedges Vegetable Frittata* plus 1 slice sprouted-grain bread and a drizzle of olive oil

LUNCH: 1 cup Beet and Orange Salad* with small 100% whole-grain roll with half of a 6-ounce can wild salmon

DINNER: 2 slices Easy Vegetable Pizza*

SNACK: 1 cup fruit salad topped with 2 tablespoons chopped walnuts *or* 2 Peanut Butter Balls*

WEEK 3

Sunday

BREAKFAST: 3 (4-inch) buckwheat pancakes (such as Bob's Red Mill), topped with ½ cup raspberries, ½ cup blueberries, and 2 teaspoons pure maple syrup

LUNCH: 1½ cups Black Bean Soup* with 8 whole-grain crackers

DINNER: a 4-ounce baked chicken breast with 1 cup roasted purple carrots (see Roasted Root Vegetables* recipe) and ½ cup cooked quinoa

SNACKS: 1 can sardines with 8 100% whole-grain crackers *or* 1 cup Roasted Beet Chips*

Monday

BREAKFAST: Spicy breakfast burrito (scramble 1 egg and 1 egg white with 3 tablespoons low-fat Cheddar cheese; place in corn tortilla with ¼ cup salsa, ¼ cup corn kernels, and a splash of hot sauce)

LUNCH: Creamy Peanut Quinoa Bowl with Sweet Potatoes*

DINNER: Salmon patty (use wild frozen variety) with a side of broccoli and ½ cup cooked brown rice

SNACK: Roasted garlic (cut the top from one head of garlic, drizzle with olive oil and roast in foil at 400°F for 25 minutes) with 6 to 8 almond meal crackers *or* as many bell pepper sticks as you'd like with ¼ cup Hummus*

Tuesday

BREAKFAST: Energizing Kale Smoothie*

LUNCH: Almond butter and raspberry sandwich (place 1 tablespoon
almond butter and ¼ cup raspberries or pear slices on 2 slices
100% whole-grain bread)

DINNER: 2 cups spaghetti squash with 1 cup no-added-sugar tomato
sauce and 3 Spinach Turkey Meatballs* (To prepare spaghetti
squash: Cut squash in half lengthwise and remove seeds; brush
the squash flesh with extra-virgin olive oil and place, face down,
on a baking pan. Bake at 400°F for 30 to 45 minutes, or until
tender; use a fork to pull out the strands.)

SNACK: A handful of pistachios with 1 small apple *or* ¼ cup dried
edamame

Wednesday

BREAKFAST: 1 cup shredded wheat cereal with 3 tablespoons walnuts,
1 tablespoon chia seeds, and ½ cup strawberries with 1 cup
unsweetened almond milk

LUNCH: 1½ cups canned low-sodium, vegetarian lentil soup with 1
cup chopped spinach added, plus a small whole-grain sourdough
roll on the side

DINNER: 4 ounces baked chicken with ½ cup cooked black bean
pasta mixed with ¼ cup jarred pesto and 1 cup Roasted Brussels
Sprouts*

SNACKS: 1 apple and 1 stick string cheese *or* 1 to 2 handfuls of dry-
roasted peanuts

Thursday

BREAKFAST: 1 cup cooked steel-cut oats with ½ cup fresh berries and
2 tablespoons walnuts

LUNCH: 4 to 5 ounces baked salmon with 1 cup steamed broccolini
and ½ cup cooked quinoa with 1 tablespoon olive oil

DINNER: 1 cup Red Lentil Soup* and ½ cup Curried Cauliflower*

SNACK: 2 Vegan Truffles* *or* celery with 2 tablespoons almond butter
and 1 tablespoon flaxseeds

Friday

BREAKFAST: 1 whole egg and 2 egg whites scrambled with ½ cup
shiitake mushrooms and ¼ onion, chopped. Serve with 1 slice
whole-grain toast or wrapped in a brown rice wrap

LUNCH: Open-faced avocado sandwich (1 slice whole-grain toast,
topped with ½ avocado, sliced, ¼ cup broccoli sprouts, and 3
tablespoons Hummus*; add ¼ cup sliced raw red onion, if desired)

DINNER: 1½ cups turmeric-rich grilled vegetables (sliced red peppers,
mushrooms, onions, zucchini, marinated in 2 tablespoons olive
oil, 1 tablespoon lemon juice, 1½ teaspoons turmeric, salt and
pepper, then grilled or broiled) served over 1 cup cooked farro

SNACK: 1 banana, smashed, with 1 tablespoon crunchy no-added-
sugar peanut butter and 1 tablespoon melted chocolate chips on
top *or* 1 cup cherries

Saturday

BREAKFAST: Pomegranate parfait (mix 1 cup low-fat plain Greek
yogurt with 1 tablespoon honey, 1 teaspoon pure vanilla extract,
and 3 tablespoons chopped pecans; add ½ cup pomegranate seeds
on top)

LUNCH: Grilled eggplant sandwich (slice eggplant into thin slices
and brush with garlic-infused olive oil, then grill it or lightly
sauté it; arrange it on 2 slices grilled sprouted-grain bread with 3
tablespoons avocado smear and ½ cup spinach)

DINNER: 2 slices Zucchini Pesto Pizza*, plus a simple green salad with
balsamic dressing for an even bigger antioxidant boost.

SNACK: 1 medium-size kiwi with 2 to 3 medium-size dried figs *or*
1 serving 100% whole-grain pretzels with ½ cup Edamame
Hummus*

WEEK 4

Sunday

BREAKFAST: Banana open-faced sandwich (cut 1 banana lengthwise,
spread 1 tablespoon almond butter on each side, add 1 teaspoon
dried cherries and 1 teaspoon hemp seeds)

LUNCH: 1 cup Blackberry Freekeh Salad* with 3 Chia Turkey Meatballs*

DINNER: 1 cup spiralized zucchini, sautéed lightly in olive oil, seasoned with salt and pepper; serve with 3 large grilled wild shrimp, topped with 1 cup arugula and a drizzle of lemon-infused olive oil.

SNACK: Baked whole apple with ground cinnamon or 1 cup Crispy Chickpeas*

Monday

BREAKFAST: 1 cup shredded wheat cereal with ¼ cup no-added-sugar coconut shreds, 3 tablespoons hemp seeds, and 1 cup unsweetened almond milk

LUNCH: 1 cup Warm Mushroom and Kale Salad* with ½ cup cubed tempeh

DINNER: 2 vegetable and shrimp kebabs (a combo of shrimp, chunks of bell pepper, tomatoes, and onion, seasoned with salt and pepper) with 1 cup cooked brown rice

SNACKS: 3½ cups plain popcorn or 1 cup mixed berries with ½ cup low-fat Greek yogurt

Tuesday

BREAKFAST: 1 cup Tropical Breakfast Bowl*

LUNCH: 1½ cups Kale and Apple Salad*

DINNER: 1 cup black bean pasta with 1 cup steamed broccolini, 1 tablespoon garlic-infused olive oil, and a 4- to 5-ounce chicken breast, grilled or baked, seasoned with salt and pepper

SNACK: ½ cup Roasted Beet Chips* or 2 Peanut Butter Balls*

Wednesday

BREAKFAST: 1 fried egg, with a 100% whole wheat English muffin, topped with 1 slice low-fat Cheddar cheese

LUNCH: 1 cup cooked lentils with a 4- to 5-ounce serving of seared wild salmon and ½ cup shredded carrots

DINNER: 1 large Cauliflower Steak* with 1 cup cubed tofu, sautéed in 1 tablespoon coconut oil, seasoned with salt and pepper

SNACK: 1 cup 100% whole wheat or spelt pretzels plus ¼ cup Hummus* or ¼ cup healthy trail mix (made with ½ cup sprouted pumpkin seeds, ½ cup raw cashews, ½ cup almonds, and ½ cup dark chocolate chips)

Thursday

BREAKFAST: 1 cup Overnight Soaked Oats*; enjoy cold or heat in microwave

LUNCH: Loaded sweet potato (microwave 1 medium-size sweet potato until cooked through; slice open and stuff with ½ cup black beans, ¼ cup low-fat Cheddar cheese, and ¼ cup Greek yogurt)

DINNER: Tuna Patty* served in a 100% whole-grain pita pocket with ½ cup broccoli sprouts; pair with 1 cup steamed broccoli

SNACK: 8 dried apricots dipped in ¼ cup melted dark chocolate or ½ cup each chopped pear and apple, dusted with ground cinnamon

Friday

BREAKFAST: 1 egg, lightly fried in 1 teaspoon olive oil, topped with ½ cup broccoli sprouts and seasoned with salt and pepper; pair with 1 to 2 slices sprouted-grain bread

LUNCH: 1 salmon patty (frozen wild-caught), cooked and served on a 100% whole-grain bun with a kale and spinach salad (top 1 cup kale and 1 cup spinach with 2 tablespoons olive oil, 2 teaspoons fig balsamic vinegar, 1 teaspoon honey, and salt and pepper)

DINNER: 3 Swiss Chard Chicken Tacos*

SNACK: 1 Pumpkin Bar* or 1 cup baked tortilla chips with ½ cup salsa

Saturday

BREAKFAST: Scrambled eggs (1 whole egg plus 2 egg whites) in a brown rice wrap with a sprinkle of low-fat Cheddar cheese

LUNCH: Creamy Peanut Quinoa Bowl with Sweet Potatoes*

DINNER: 1 cup edamame pasta with 1 cup no-added-sugar tomato sauce, 3 tablespoons Parmesan cheese, and 1 cup steamed broccoli

SNACK: 1 hard-boiled egg with ½ avocado, sliced, and a light drizzle of olive oil, seasoned with salt and pepper, or 1 cup low-fat yogurt with ½ cup blackberries and 1 teaspoon honey

chapter 10

The Skinny Liver Diet

IF YOU WANT TO LOSE WEIGHT, you've come to the right place—er, chapter! I'm not going to lie to you, though: Losing weight isn't easy, as many of my patients know all too well. But it doesn't have to be as hard as it seems, either. The process of slimming down can fall somewhere between the two ends of the spectrum, in the gray zone, but only *if* you develop the right mind-set. To shed pounds and keep them off, you'll need to change your eating habits, but you'll also need to alter your behavior in other areas of your life. That's the key to lasting weight-loss success—and I promise: *you* can find that key and put it to good work to unlock better health for yourself. In my work, I have helped countless people lose weight and enhance their health, and I'm going to help you do that, too.

It's worth the effort because shedding excess weight has so many positive ripple effects—for your liver, your heart, your brain, and pretty much every other part of you. If you're overweight, a reduction in weight, even a small one, can lead to big benefits to your liver, reducing liver inflammation, the buildup of scar tissue (fibrosis) and fatty deposits, and alleviating insulin resistance and other markers of metabolic syndrome; these latter conditions play supporting roles in nonalcoholic fatty liver disease (NAFLD). As you now know, two of the best ways to reverse fatty liver disease are through diet and exercise changes that lead to weight loss. In fact, research has found that among people with NAFLD, losing weight can lead to the complete disappearance of NAFLD. Slimming down is really *that* powerful!

On a basic physiological level, weight loss involves nothing more than taking in fewer calories from food than you expend through normal bodily functions and physical activities. The balance of these influences simply needs to fall to the right side of the fulcrum (more calories are burned than are consumed) for weight-loss to occur. If the balance shifts to the wrong side (too many calories are consumed and too few are burned), the excess calories are stored as fat, which is bad news for your liver and your waistline!

To take the steady, sustainable approach to losing weight, I recommend aiming for a calorie deficit of 500 calories per day. This will allow you to lose at least 1 pound per week (since a pound of body fat is equal to 3,500 calories), which is a steady, sustainable rate of weight loss. You can do this by cutting 500 calories from your daily diet, burning an extra 500 extra calories a day through exercise, or taking the combination approach by trimming 250 calories from your food intake and torching an extra 250 through physical activity. My opinion is the latter approach is best because: (a) making a 250-calorie reduction in your food intake isn't as jarring to the system as a 500-calorie one is; and (b) incorporating exercise into your regimen helps prevent muscle loss and it provides added protective perks to your liver and cardiovascular system, as previously described. The good news is that you don't need to count calories; I've done that for you in this plan!

The following weight-loss plan will provide you with 1,200 to 1,600 calories a day, which will help you achieve lasting weight loss without causing you to feel deprived. If you aim to lose a pound per week and set reasonable, attainable long-term goals, you'll be setting yourself up for success. So, if your big-picture goal is to shed 40 pounds, a good approach is to strive to lose 10 pounds in the next two months, then hit Repeat and strive for the next milestone (another ten) from there. In fact, research suggests that people who lose weight gradually and steadily are better able to keep it off over the long haul. Once you reach your goal weight, you'll want to return to "The Love-Your-Liver Eating Plan" (see Chapter 9) for lifelong maintenance.

After years of seeing people struggle with their weight-loss goals, I have gained valuable perspective on strategies that can help make the process of losing weight easier. Believe it or not, it's often the little things that thwart people's weight-loss goals, whether it's their usual (high-fat, high-calorie) sandwich spread, condiments that make meals tastier, a habit of drinking too many calories, waiting too long to snack between meals, or other factors. I have incorporated these insights into this plan so that you won't have to think about them.

Besides containing a reduction in calories (from what you're consuming now), this weight-loss plan contains lots of probiotic-rich foods, antioxidant-rich fruits and veggies, fiber-filled whole grains, and anti-inflammatory omega-3 fatty acids (fish lovers, rejoice!). It's devoid of proinflammatory foods (such as simple sugars, refined or stripped carbs, most saturated fats, and trans fats) that harm the liver and various aspects of cardiovascular health, and it contains foods that help regulate blood sugar levels and lipid control, which is significant because reducing risk factors for cardiovascular disease and diabetes tends to go hand in hand with boosting liver health. You'll find moderate amounts of healthy fats (in the form of nuts and olive oil, in particular) and health-promoting herbs and spices to keep your meals delicious and nutritious. All of these approaches are designed to improve the condition of your liver while helping you slim down, which will in turn enhance the well-being of this vital organ.

After getting divorced, Melissa, 67, was ready to lose weight (she carried 20 extra pounds, mostly around her midsection) and get on with her life, which is why she came to see me a couple of years ago. A mother of five grown children, she had a rigorous volunteer schedule with various nonprofit organizations. Melissa's diet depended on her freezer and microwave for the first few meals of the day and special events catering for the evening meals. Aside from doing yoga once in a while, she didn't exercise or do much to manage her stress. She also consumed alcohol at least five nights a week at events.

To help her slim down, I encouraged her to start eating real foods (instead of frozen meals) and helped her figure out how to navigate a special-events menu so she could get the healthiest meals possible. The first thing Melissa did was to take a healthy cooking class. Gradually, she shifted to a more plant-based diet, filled with colorful fruits and vegetables, fiber, healthy fats, and free of additives and preservatives. Through the cooking class, she met women who were runners, and within a few months, Melissa ran her first 5k race. She also began tracking her meals with a smart phone.

HOT TIPS!

Here are some useful strategies that can help you stay on track with your plan:

Confide in those you trust: Tell your closest circle of family members and friends about your health-promoting, weight-loss goals and ask them to support you on the journey and help you avoid temptations that you want to resist. If you can tell them specifically how they can help you (say, by not bringing you sweet treats), that's even better. Hopefully, this proactive request will ward off inadvertent sabotage from other people.

Drink a tall glass of water before meals: You probably know that consuming thick liquids like soup or vegetable juice before a meal can help curb your food intake during the meal—but water can, too. A 2010 study from Virginia Tech found that when overweight adults drank 16 ounces of water before each meal, they consumed fewer calories from their meals and lost 44 percent more weight after twelve weeks than did their counterparts who didn't drink up. This may be because consuming water before a meal decreases sensations of hunger and increases feelings of fullness, the researchers note.

Remind yourself this isn't your last chance to eat: If you find yourself wanting to continue eating but you think you've actually had enough at a meal, hit the Pause button. Your brain may not have caught up with your stomach and registered fullness; many people eat so quickly that they miss out on their body's satiety cues. Do something else for a while and check in with yourself: If you're still hungry in, say, an hour, have a small, healthy snack.

After working with me for six months, her cholesterol level had gone down, her hemoglobin A1C (a marker of blood sugar management) level had decreased, and she had lost 27 pounds. She looked amazing—and said she felt like "a stronger, healthier, more vibrant version" of herself. An inspiring success story, Melissa credits her weight loss and transformation to finally learning how to eat and cook healthfully, dine out smartly, and gain valuable support from health-conscious friends.

What follows is a four-week plan that's designed to help you lose weight and prevent or reverse NAFLD. Here are some guidelines to keep in mind while looking at the menu plans:

- **Protein provides the centerpiece of every breakfast.** Protein-rich foods—such as eggs, low-fat dairy products (yogurt, for example), and tofu but not processed meats—are an important part of breakfast for several reasons: They are easy to make, they are chock-full of nutrients (such as choline in eggs; after all, deficiencies of choline in the body have been shown to cause adverse effects on the liver), and they are filling and satisfying, which makes them helpful for blood sugar control. Several studies have shown that having eggs in the morning may help in the battle against the bulge and may also help you resist cravings for junk food later in the day. (By the way, there's no reason to avoid eating eggs regularly because they don't seem to cause adverse effects to your cholesterol as we all once thought; it's now known that saturated fat and trans fats are the dietary culprits that raise blood cholesterol.) Other studies suggest that having protein at breakfast can help you succeed at losing weight.

- **The Skinny Liver Diet is low in sugar and devoid of refined grains.** All the foods you'll enjoy on this plan are whole, as unprocessed as they come. Given that, resist the urge to add sugar or artificial sweeteners to some of the items here (such as coffee or yogurt). This principle also applies to items you might have to buy, such as peanut butter (read the label and make sure sugar hasn't been added). This is one reason the plan doesn't allow unnaturally fat-free products (such as fat-free salad dressing, pudding, or cookies), which are often swimming in sugar to make up for the flavor that's lost from eliminating fat. This plan will help you eliminate excessive sugar and train your taste buds and brain to no longer want or need it.

- **Season your food with liver-boosting herbs and spices.** These are incorporated into many recipes and it's fine to add more delicious herbs, roots, and spices, such as thyme, rosemary, cumin, oregano, cilantro, chives, parsley, basil, ginger, cinnamon, and garlic at your discretion. Keep in mind: Curcumin (found in turmeric) may prevent or treat liver damage from advanced forms of fatty liver disease, according to research from Saint Louis University. Consuming cinnamon appears to decrease cholesterol abnormalities, inflammatory markers, and elevated liver en-zymes in people with NAFLD, according to research from Iran. And piperine, a component of black pepper, may prevent the for-mation of new fat cells, which will benefit your liver and the rest of you, so feel free to add these to your food.

- **Allow yourself a cheat-meal.** But don't let it turn into a cheat-weekend. When you're trying to lose weight, it's important to maintain consistency in your eating habits, but it's okay to splurge once in a while. I tell my patients there's nothing wrong with having a cheat-meal once a week where they can consume whatever they want but still in a reasonable portion. One of my patients has a cheeseburger and fries every Saturday night, while another chooses to have a small hot fudge sundae on Fri-days with her son. Building these pleasant indulgences into your plan may actually help to keep you on track for the long haul.

- **Slow yourself down.** By chewing your food thoroughly and put-ting your fork down between bites, you'll naturally eat more slowly, giving your stomach sufficient time to send a message to the brain that it's had enough. This way, you'll consume fewer calories and gain plenty of satisfaction. Your gut will have am-ple time to secrete the hormones ghrelin and leptin, which send signals of hunger and fullness to your brain—before you have eaten too much. I often ask my patients how they know when to stop eating, and the most common answers are *when the food on my plate is gone* or *when I'm stuffed.* A healthier approach is to eat until you are no longer hungry, rather than truly full—a tac-tic that will have a positive effect on your weight. Chewing your food slowly and pausing between bites will help you get there.

- **Think about your drinks.** Consume lots of water and calorie-free beverages (such as seltzer with a wedge of lemon or lime or iced tea), as well as hot tea and coffee if you enjoy these beverages. In moderation, coffee is particularly beneficial to the liver and can help reduce inflammation. All of these beverages can help you shed unwanted pounds because they're calorie-free as long as you don't add sweeteners.

COPING WITH CRAVINGS

When cravings for a particular food (usually sweet or salty items) strike, people often think it's a sign that their body needs that particular food or taste. But that's not true. It simply means your mind or your mouth wants that particular item for psychological reasons. To prevent cravings from sabotaging your slim-down efforts, eat whole foods regularly to keep your hunger in check around the clock and stay well hydrated.

When cravings do occur, build in a pause to see whether they pass naturally and engage in an engrossing activity in the meantime. If your craving just won't quit, try substituting a healthy choice: To satisfy a sweet craving, have a bowl of juicy mango chunks; to quench your desire for something salty, a cup of miso soup may do the trick. If your craving is undeniably for chocolate, you might have a small piece of chocolate bark, a vegan truffle, or a couple of cinnamon baked almonds (which contain cocoa powder)—and savor the flavor. Then, call it quits!

- **Eat every 4 hours.** Whether it's a meal or a snack, having something to eat every 4 hours helps you maintain steady blood sugar levels and helps you avoid getting overly hungry and overeating later. The reason nutrition experts warn against going out to dinner, a movie, or the grocery store on an empty stomach is because hunger is powerful: It can cause you to reach for starchy or sugary foods that will bump up your blood sugar and make you feel good almost immediately due to that rapid rise in blood sugar; moments of intense hunger rarely lead you to stuff your face with broccoli. Part of a good weight-management plan is to avoid setting yourself up for extreme hunger.
- **Pump up the volume.** Loading up on vegetables, fruit, whole grains, and lean proteins will help you eat less by filling you up with a greater volume of food. Items that contain a substantial amount of water (such as soups) or air (such as smoothies) will do the same thing. This principle is an essential part of this weight-loss plan, which provides foods that fill you up.
- **Give yourself a 5-minute breather.** Sometimes, a timer is all you need to end a craving since many cravings pass in 5 to 10

minutes. So if you set a timer for that amount of time and distract yourself in the meantime—by folding laundry, catching up on personal e-mails, organizing recent photos, or completing another task—there's a good chance your yen for cookies, chips, or something else will dissipate by the time the buzzer goes off. [See box on previous page for more tips on managing cravings.]

- **Say good-bye to bad habits for good.** It's true that old habits may die hard, but it's essential to put them in the grave if you want to lose weight once and for all. In a study published in a 2011 issue of the *New England Journal of Medicine*, researchers from Harvard Medical School found that people were most likely to gain small amounts of weight over the years if they increased their consumption of potato chips and sugar-sweetened beverages, decreased their physical activity, increased how much time they spent watching television, and got either too much sleep (more than 8 hours a night) or too little sleep (fewer than 6 hours). Most alarmingly, researchers found that people could start seeing changes in their weight within only months of adopting these harmful behaviors. The bottom line: If you want to keep the excess weight off for good, don't let bad habits slip back into your routine.

Savvy Portion-Control Strategies

Upgrading your diet and losing weight aren't just about what you choose to eat. These goals also require that you pay attention to portion sizes. It's no secret that we live in an age where portion distortion is common but that doesn't mean you have to succumb to this pattern. Here are five ways to avoid it for the sake of your waistline and your liver.

Downsize your plates and bowls Brian Wansink, PhD, and his colleagues at Cornell University have done extensive research on how the size of the plate influences how much people eat and how well they control their portions. They have found, again and again, that the bigger the plate, the more food people are likely to put on it and the more they're likely to eat. Swapping your entrée plates for smaller salad plates can work wonders when it comes to satisfying your eyes and your stomach. The same is true of replacing giant bowls with smaller ones.

Visualize real-life portion proportions Since it's not realistic to carry around measuring cups and spoons, it helps to picture what a proper portion should look like in relation to everyday objects. Some examples: A serving of fish is about the size of a checkbook; a serving of meat or chicken resembles a deck of cards or your palm; a proper portion of rice, pasta, legumes, and vegetables is about the size of your fist; a serving of fruit is about the size of a tennis ball; 2 tablespoons of peanut butter is the size of a Ping-Pong ball; and a serving of oil is the size of your thumb.

Invest in plastic sandwich bags Rather than eating foods that come in a big box directly from the box, divvy up portions of cereal or whole-grain crackers or pretzels into resealable plastic sandwich bags, then put these in a shoebox in the pantry. Just seeing how much a portion is, as opposed to mindless grabbing from the bag, will help you keep your intake of snacklike items under control. Of course, you could also buy items in single-serving bags, but you'll pay more for the convenience of going the prepackaged route.

Snack on foods you have to work harder to get in your mouth Noshing on peanuts or pistachios that come in the shell, popcorn kernels that you've cooked on the stove instead of the microwave, and foods that need to be peeled and/or cut up (an orange or mango, for instance) eliminates opportunities for mindless eating. Plus, the work of having to make these items ready to pop in your mouth naturally slows down the eating process, which in turn helps curb your intake.

Avoid a family-style setup. Rather than placing serving dishes on the table, keep them on the stove or kitchen counter. Put your meal on plates there, then bring the plates to the table. It's a simple adjustment that helps you control your intake and discourages you from mindlessly reaching for second helpings just because the food is on the table. If you feel the need to have something on the table, make it a salad or a nonstarchy vegetable (such as steamed broccoli or asparagus) since it's hard to eat too much of these foods (given how filling and relatively low in calories they are). If you want to take things a step further (and avoid the temptation of nibbling from the pots and pans), you can quickly store the leftovers in the fridge for another day.

The Four-Week Meal Plan

Without further ado, here's a four-week meal plan that will show your liver the love it deserves while helping you lose weight. Bon appétit!

Note: You'll find that all the recipes in the plan below with an * are marked ⑤ in Appendix A at the back of the book.

WEEK 1

Sunday

BREAKFAST: Crustless Quiche Cups* with ¼ cup chopped leek and ¼ cup chopped sun-dried tomatoes

SNACK: 6 whole walnuts and 1 orange

LUNCH: Greek salad (2 cups dark leafy greens, 3 chopped olives, ¼ cup chopped tomato, ¼ cup chopped cucumber, 1 tablespoon feta cheese, and 2 tablespoons balsamic dressing), topped with 4 ounces grilled chicken strips

DINNER: Cauliflower-Crust Pizza* with 1 cup no-added-sugar tomato sauce and 1 cup chopped spinach

SNACK OR TREAT: ½ cup wild blueberries with 1 cup low-fat Greek yogurt

Monday

BREAKFAST: 1 hard-boiled egg, chopped, and 1 slice avocado, wrapped in a brown rice tortilla or wrap

SNACK: 1 medium-size apple and 1 tablespoon no-added-sugar peanut butter

LUNCH: ¼ cup Hummus* with 3 whole carrots and ½ turkey sandwich on whole-grain bread (4 ounces turkey, 3 avocado slices, 1 slice tomato)

DINNER: 4 ounces grilled salmon with 1 cup steamed garlicky broccoli and ½ cup cooked quinoa

SNACK OR TREAT: ½ grapefruit and 1 ounce (a small handful) almonds

Tuesday

BREAKFAST: ½ cup old-fashioned oats, cooked in unsweetened almond milk, topped with 2 tablespoons slivered almonds and ¼ cup blackberries

SNACK: ½ cup wild blueberries and 1 cup plain low-fat yogurt with 1 teaspoon ground cinnamon

LUNCH: Zucchini and Farro Salad* with 3 large grilled shrimp on top

DINNER: 4 ounces grass-fed lean hamburger, in a wrap made of mustard greens, with ½ cup Sweet Potato Fries* (about 8)

SNACK OR TREAT: ½ cup Overnight Chia Seed Pudding*

Wednesday

BREAKFAST: 3 scrambled egg whites with 2 tablespoons canned jalapeño peppers and ½ cup salsa

SNACK: 1 ounce (a handful) of pistachios

LUNCH: 4 ounces turkey breast with 2 cups arugula, ¼ cup celery, 2 tablespoons dried cranberries, 1 teaspoon lemon juice, 1 tablespoon extra-virgin olive oil, and 2 whole-grain breadsticks or 4 whole-grain melba toasts

DINNER: 1½ cups Chickpea Stew* with a side of 1 cup steamed Swiss chard, and 4 whole wheat pita wedges (1 small pita sliced into 4 wedges)

SNACK OR TREAT: ¼ cup trail mix (a blend of sunflower seeds, almonds, and dried apricots, chopped up)

Thursday

BREAKFAST: 1 slice whole-grain toast, topped with 1 tablespoon almond butter, ½ cup sliced strawberries on the side

SNACK: ¼ cup Hummus* with ½ cup red pepper sticks

LUNCH: 2 cups baby spinach salad with 4 ounces pan-seared tempeh and 1 tablespoon basil-flavored extra-virgin olive oil

DINNER: Stir-fry made with 2 tablespoons minced garlic,

2 tablespoons minced ginger, ½ cup cubed tofu, ½ cup snow peas, ½ cup shredded carrot, over ½ cup cooked brown rice

SNACK OR TREAT: ½ cup raspberries with 1 tablespoon 70% cacao dark chocolate chips

Friday

BREAKFAST: Protein smoothie, made with no-added-sugar protein powder (such as Orgain chocolate), ½ banana, 1 cup almond milk, and ice

SNACK: ½ cup steamed edamame

LUNCH: ½ cup Chicken Salad* on 1 brown rice cake with ½ cup fruit salad

DINNER: 1 serving Herb-Roasted Salmon with Brussels Sprouts*

SNACK OR TREAT: 4 Medjool dates

Saturday

BREAKFAST: Red pepper and zucchini, egg white frittata (made with 3 egg whites, ½ cup diced red bell pepper, ½ cup chopped zucchini)

SNACK: 2 whole celery sticks with 1 tablespoon nut butter, sprinkled with 1 teaspoon flaxseeds

LUNCH: 1 vegetarian burger on top of 2 cups spinach salad, with ¼ cup blackberries, ¼ cup raspberries, and 2 tablespoons lemon-infused olive oil mixed with 1 tablespoon balsamic vinegar

DINNER: 4 ounces grilled tuna steak with ½ cup steamed broccoli and ½ cup pearled whole-grain couscous

SNACK OR TREAT: 3 cups SkinnyPop popcorn

WEEK 2

Sunday

BREAKFAST: Tofu scramble (made with ½ cup extra-firm, cubed tofu and ½ cup scrambled egg whites, sautéed in 1 tablespoon olive oil and seasoned with ground turmeric); ½ cup blueberries on the side

SNACK: 1 medium-size apple with 1 tablespoon no-added-sugar peanut butter

LUNCH: 1½ cups Miso Soup with Spinach and Tofu*, plus 3 to 4 strips
  seaweed with ½ cup Asian snap peas and carrots
DINNER: 1 cup Chicken and Broccoli Pad Thai*
SNACK OR TREAT: ¼ cup Crispy Chickpeas*

Monday
BREAKFAST: Veggie basil omelet (1 whole egg, 1 egg white, ½ cup
  chopped tomato, ½ cup chopped basil, ¼ cup low-fat cottage
  cheese); ½ pear
SNACK: 1½ cups "cheesy" popcorn (sprinkled with nutritional yeast)
LUNCH: ½ cup Albacore Tuna Salad* on 1 brown rice cake, small side
  salad with balsamic vinegar
DINNER: 1 cup 3-Bean Chili* sprinkled with 2 tablespoons low-fat
  Cheddar cheese
SNACK OR TREAT: ½ banana dipped in 1 tablespoon melted chocolate
  chips

Tuesday
BREAKFAST: Smoothie bowl (made with 1 cup low-fat plain yogurt, ¼
  cup blueberries, ¼ cup raspberries, and 2 tablespoons chopped
  walnuts)
SNACK: 1 cup wild blueberries
LUNCH: 1 cup Apple, Pear, and Jicama Waldorf Salad*, with 1 cup Easy
  Corn Soup*
DINNER: 4 ounces Salmon Arlene* with 6 pieces broccolini, drizzled
  with 1 teaspoon extra virgin olive oil, ½ cup cooked brown rice
SNACK OR TREAT: 1 small package (0.35 ounces) roasted seaweed snacks

Wednesday
BREAKFAST: 1 hard-boiled egg, drizzled with 1 teaspoon olive oil,
  pepper, 1 slice toasted sprouted-grain bread with 1 slice avocado
  spread on it; 1 mandarin orange
SNACK: 1 Peanut Butter Ball*
LUNCH: 2 cups arugula with ¼ cup shaved Parmesan cheese, 2
  tablespoons dried cherries, 2 tablespoons pistachios, and 1
  tablespoon lemon-infused extra-virgin olive oil

DINNER: 1 cup Thai Peanut Spaghetti Squash* with 4 strips grilled
chicken breast on satay-style skewers

SNACK OR TREAT: ½ grapefruit

Thursday

BREAKFAST: Quick omelet (made with 3 egg whites and 2 tablespoons
low-fat Cheddar cheese, cooked for 1 minute in the microwave in a
ramekin cup)

SNACK: 6 whole walnuts

LUNCH: 1 tuna patty over 1 cup steamed spinach, ½ cup fruit salad

DINNER: 1 cup Root Vegetable Gratin* with 2 cups arugula drizzled
with 2 tablespoons lemon-infused extra-virgin olive oil

SNACK OR TREAT: ½ cup Overnight Chia Seed Pudding* with ¼ cup
blackberries

Friday

BREAKFAST: 1 hard-boiled egg with 1 cup old-fashioned oats topped
with ½ cup chopped apple and ½ cup raspberries

SNACK: 8 flaxseed crackers with 1 tablespoon almond butter

LUNCH: 2 cups Crispy Chickpea Salad* with 2 tablespoons balsamic
vinaigrette

DINNER: 4 ounces Spicy Turkey Burger* with 10 spears grilled
asparagus

SNACK OR TREAT: ½ cup Chocolate Espresso Tofu Mousse*

Saturday

BREAKFAST: 2 (4-inch) protein-rich pancakes (made with no-added-sugar
buckwheat pancake mix such as Bob's Red Mill), with 1 tablespoon
pea protein powder added), topped with ½ cup raspberries

SNACK: 1 ounce (a handful) of pistachios

LUNCH: 4 ounces Chicken Salad* in ½ whole wheat pita, with 1 cup
steamed broccoli

DINNER: 4 ounces baked trout with 1 cup Roasted Brussels Sprouts*
and 1 medium-size baked sweet potato

SNACK OR TREAT: ½ cup raspberries mixed with 1 tablespoon chopped
walnuts and 1 teaspoon melted dark chocolate

WEEK 3

Sunday

BREAKFAST: 1 egg, cooked over easy, with 1 cup wilted garlic spinach, wrapped with 1 slice low-fat Cheddar cheese in a brown rice wrap or tortilla

SNACK: 1 cup low-fat Greek yogurt with ½ cup bananas and ground cinnamon

LUNCH: 1 cup low-fat cottage cheese, ½ apple (diced), ½ cup pineapple, ¼ cup walnuts, ground cinnamon

DINNER: Portobello Mushroom Sandwich*, ½ cup Sweet Potato Fries* (about 8)

SNACK OR TREAT: 1 ounce (1 handful) Cinnamon Baked Almonds*

Monday

BREAKFAST: 2 Veggie Quinoa Quiche Cups*

SNACK: 1 medium-size apple plus 1 tablespoon no-added-sugar peanut butter

LUNCH: 4 ounces grilled chicken with 2 cups romaine salad, ½ cup blueberries, cherry tomatoes, and lemon-infused olive oil

DINNER: 3 Chia Turkey Meatballs* with ½ cup black-bean pasta, ½ cup no-added-sugar marinara sauce, and a mixed green salad on the side

SNACK OR TREAT: 1 small baked apple, sprinkled with ground cinnamon

Tuesday

BREAKFAST: 3 slices smoked salmon on top of 1 whole wheat bagel thin, with 1 tablespoon low-fat cream cheese

SNACK: 6 to 10 whole-grain crackers with 2 tablespoons black bean hummus

LUNCH: 1 cup Butternut Squash Soup*, topped with ½ cup cooked quinoa and ½ cup wilted spinach

DINNER: 1 Salmon Cake* with 2 cups mesclun mix salad with 2 tablespoons balsamic vinaigrette

SNACK OR TREAT: 3 cups air-popped popcorn

Wednesday

BREAKFAST: 2 eggs scrambled with 1 ½ teaspoons ground turmeric in
   1 teaspoon extra-virgin olive oil

SNACK: 1 cup low-fat cottage cheese with ½ cup cubed peach

LUNCH: 1 cup cooked steel-cut oatmeal with ½ cup chopped apple and
   1 teaspoon ground cinnamon

DINNER: 4 ounces broiled grass-fed flank steak, with 1 cup roasted
   cauliflower and 1 cup steamed broccoli

SNACK OR TREAT: 2 Medjool dates stuffed with 1 teaspoon no-added-
   sugar peanut butter

Thursday

BREAKFAST: Overnight Chia Seed Pudding*, topped with ¼ cup
   chopped pecans and ¼ cup chopped dried apricots (may add 1
   tablespoon honey for sweetness, if desired)

SNACK: ¼ cup Edamame Hummus* with 12 baked tortilla chips

LUNCH: Half of a 6-ounce can of wild salmon atop 1 cup Kale Pesto
   and Barley Salad*

DINNER: 1½ cups Miso Soup with Spinach and Tofu*, with 2 Brown
   Rice Balls*

SNACK OR TREAT: 1 ounce Chocolate Bark*

Friday

BREAKFAST: 1 poached egg, 2 ounces smoked salmon on 1 brown rice
   cake

SNACK: 1 cup Warm Mushroom and Kale Salad*

LUNCH: 1 cup Broccoli Salad*, topped with 1 tablespoon pumpkin
   seeds

DINNER: ½ cup black beans with 1 cup cooked quinoa and ½ cup
   avocado chunks, topped with 1 teaspoon extra-virgin olive oil

SNACK OR TREAT: 1 orange

Saturday

BREAKFAST: Protein-packed kale smoothie (made with 1 cup shredded
   kale, 1 chopped apple, 1 cup chopped cucumber, 1 scoop plain pea
   protein powder)

SNACK: 5 sardines on 5 to 6 100% whole-grain crackers

LUNCH: 1 cup Mango Quinoa Salad* with a side of 8 to 12 baked
    tortilla chips and ½ cup salsa

DINNER: 1 cup curried Tofu, Cashew, and Broccoli Stir-fry* on top of
    ½ cup cooked black rice

SNACK OR TREAT: ½ cup Overnight Chia Seed Pudding

WEEK 4

Sunday

BREAKFAST: 1 slice French toast (1 slice whole-grain, gluten-free bread,
    dipped in 1 egg and sprinkled with ground cinnamon), cooked on
    a nonstick pan, topped with ½ cup sliced strawberries

SNACK: ½ cup watermelon

LUNCH: Peanut butter and banana wrap (1 brown rice wrap with 1
    tablespoon no-added-sugar peanut butter and ½ sliced banana,
    rolled up)

DINNER: 1 cup Wild Shrimp and Black Bean Salad* with 1 cup steamed
    broccoli

SNACK OR TREAT: ½ cup Chocolate Espresso Tofu Mousse*

Monday

BREAKFAST: 1 scrambled egg with 1 slice sprouted-grain toast,
    smeared with avocado

SNACK: 1 medium-size apple with 1 tablespoon no-added-sugar peanut
    butter

LUNCH: 1½ cups Roasted Beet Salad*

DINNER: 4 ounces grilled tuna steak with 2 cups spinach sautéed with
    chopped garlic, 1 cup cooked farro with 1 tablespoon garlicky
    extra-virgin olive oil

SNACK OR TREAT: 6 whole walnuts and 4 apricots

Tuesday

BREAKFAST: 1 peanut butter roll-up (made with 1 tablespoon no-added-
    sugar peanut butter, 1 sliced banana, 1 teaspoon honey, and 1
    brown rice wrap)

SNACK: ¼ cup Black Bean Hummus* and 2 medium-size spelt pretzels

LUNCH: 1 cup Curried Lentils* with ½ cup diced red pepper

DINNER: 4 ounces Sesame Seed–Crusted Tofu* with ½ cup Seaweed Salad* and 1 vegetable spring roll

SNACK OR TREAT: 1 small apple and 1 tablespoon no-added-sugar peanut butter

Wednesday

BREAKFAST: Cheesy egg wrap (1 egg white scrambled with 2 tablespoons low-fat Cheddar cheese, tucked into ½ whole-grain pita)

SNACK: 1 cup Greek low-fat yogurt with ½ cup fresh raspberries

LUNCH: 1 cup Shaved Brussels Sprouts Salad* with a vegetarian burger on a whole-grain bun

DINNER: 1 medium-size sweet potato stuffed with ½ cup cooked ground turkey and ½ cup steamed broccoli

SNACK OR TREAT: 1 ounce Cinnamon Baked Almonds*

Thursday

BREAKFAST: Steel-cut oatmeal (made with ½ cup oats cooked in 1 cup unsweetened almond milk), topped with ½ cup sliced fresh strawberries

SNACK: 2 cups air-popped popcorn

LUNCH: 1 cup Butternut Squash Soup*, topped with ½ cup whole-grain croutons or 6 large whole-grain crackers

DINNER: 4 ounces grilled or baked chicken breast on top of 1 cup roasted green beans and cauliflower, seasoned with 1½ teaspoons ground turmeric, with ½ cup cooked brown rice

SNACK OR TREAT: ½ grapefruit

Friday

BREAKFAST: Southwestern tofu scramble (½ cup cubed tofu, 1 whole egg, scrambled with ½ chopped red bell pepper and turmeric), wrapped in a brown rice wrap

SNACK: Apple and 1 tablespoon no-added-sugar peanut butter

LUNCH: 1 cup cubed pan-seared tofu on top of 1 cup Broccoli Salad*

DINNER: 4 ounces grilled salmon with 1 cup steamed green beans, 1 small whole-grain roll

SNACK OR TREAT: Chocolate-covered walnuts (6 whole walnuts dipped in ½ ounce melted dark chocolate chips)

Saturday

BREAKFAST: Apple cinnamon parfait (made with 1 cup plain, low-fat yogurt, 1 teaspoon pure vanilla extract, ½ cup chopped apple, 2 tablespoons pecans, and 1 teaspoon ground cinnamon)

SNACK: ½ cup mixed berries sprinkled with 2 tablespoons slivered almonds

LUNCH: ½ cup albacore tuna on 7 100% whole wheat or gluten-free crackers, small side salad

DINNER: Mini spinach marinara pizzas (2 halves of a 100% whole wheat English muffin, toasted and topped with no-added-sugar tomato sauce, baby spinach leaves, and a sprinkling of mozzarella cheese), with a small side salad with 2 tablespoons balsamic vinaigrette

SNACK OR TREAT: 1 Peanut Butter Ball*

Sometimes, even the best-laid plans can fail if you don't have the proper supporting tools at your disposal. To set the stage for your weight-loss plan to succeed and help you get to the prize of a slimmer you more smoothly, here are some tools that can make upgrading your eating and exercise habits easier:

- *An accurate scale:* Weigh in at least once a week. To accurately track your weight-loss progress, make friends with your scale. Getting on the scale once a week helps you catch sneaky increases in weight (that you can jump on and fix), and it can motivate you to keep up the good work when you see the results of the changes you've been making. A 2014 study from Finland found that when people who were trying to improve their health weighed themselves daily, they lost weight, whereas they tended to gain weight when they took breaks from weighing in that lasted longer than a month. A tape measure is also handy for monitoring changes in your waist and hip circumference.

- *A stress-management tip sheet:* Finding effective ways to ease stress is an essential part of succeeding at losing weight because when you're stressed out, your body's levels of cortisol (a stress hormone) rise, which in turn promotes weight gain, especially around your midsection. So if you're trying to slim down while letting stress get the upper hand, you're working at cross-purposes to your goals. The first step is to identify your stress triggers (you'll find a Stress-Trigger Tracking Sheet in Appendix B); the next is to arm yourself with tools that effectively ease your stress. As Dan Buettner, author of *The Blue Zones,* notes, the world's longest-living people have found ways to "down shift" and shed their stress: "Okinawans take a few moments each day to remember their ancestors, Adventists pray, Ikarians take a nap, and Sardinians do happy hour." Make a list of strategies that work for you— whether it's taking a luxurious bubble bath, playing with your beloved dog, listening to calming music, taking a walk in nature, or something else—and post it in a visible place in your home. Your state of mind and your body (including your liver) will appreciate the reminder.

- *An activity tracker:* Keeping track of how many steps you take in a day motivates you to take more of them, according to research from the University of Michigan. You can use a simple pedometer or a more complicated device that tracks your mileage and sleep patterns as well. Whichever route you choose, wear your activity tracker regularly and input the data to your weight-loss smartphone app (my favorite is the Lose It! app) to get more positive reinforcement to keep moving. Over the years, studies have found that continuous self-monitoring (of eating and exercise habits) helps people lose excess weight and keep it off. You'll also find a Healthy Liver Weekly Journal in Appendix C, to help you keep tabs on what you're doing, challenges you're encountering, and what you could do differently.

chapter 11

Putting the Pieces Together

AFTER FIVE YEARS OF MARRIAGE, Nathan, 40, a hardworking lawyer and father of two, had gained so much weight that he had to buy pants that were two sizes larger. He always felt hungry and his cravings were out of control. Nathan was burning the candle at both ends, often working until one a.m. and waking up at six a.m. to make it to the firm at a respectable time. When he came to see me, his LDL (the "bad") cholesterol was slightly elevated and his HDL (the "good") cholesterol was too low; this worried him because his father had died of a heart attack in his early 50s. Most of all, Nathan wanted to get a grip on his hunger, improve his eating habits, and regain his energy because he was feeling wiped out.

The first steps were to upgrade his grain choices (replacing white grains with whole grains), cut out red meat, and switch from regular sodas to naturally flavored seltzer. Nathan also began walking at least three days a week. After making these changes, his energy began to increase and his weight came down a little but his ravenous hunger and cravings were still there. After taking a deeper look at his sleep habits, I urged Nathan to make it a priority to get at least seven hours of sleep per night, since insufficient sleep can wreak havoc on hormone levels in ways that increase hunger. Once he began doing that, he lost the rest of the excess weight and his heart-disease risk factors went down, too.

As Nathan discovered, making multiple lifestyle improvements often packs a more powerful punch than adopting any single measure on its own. In his case, the combination of a more wholesome diet, regular exercise, and better sleep added up to greater health benefits, a healthier weight, and more energy, something he wasn't able to achieve just by changing his diet. As you begin to follow a liver-protective diet and exercise plan, you'll also want to engage in other ways of supporting the health of this essential organ and your overall well-being.

In other words, it's time to put together a complete liver-protection plan that's likely to work for you personally. To set the wheels of change in motion, here is a four-week calendar with "to-do" lists for how to put the different elements together that will create a healthy lifestyle for *your* liver today, tomorrow, and the foreseeable future. To help you fine-tune the process, use the Healthy Liver Journal in Appendix C.

Week 1: Start Moving!

Research shows that regular exercise plays an important role in healing your liver, and various types of exercise may help in different ways. This week will focus on getting you ready and motivated to dive into a physical activity plan that will benefit your liver, one small step at a time.

Day 1: Get clearance Find out whether you're physically ready and able to start an exercise program by getting a complete examination from your doctor. Be sure to bring any ongoing health concerns or forms of chronic pain to your doctor's attention and ask whether there are any restrictions on the types of activities you can do, based on these issues. If you don't get the green light to exercise right away, find out what you need to do to get it.

Day 2: Redefine "exercise" If you don't like formal gym workouts or hardcore sweat-fests, make a list of physical activities you do enjoy, such as dancing, gardening, walking, riding your bike, or doing something else. The right exercise for you is the one you'll actually do on a regular basis, not necessarily the one your best friend or neighbor swears by. It also helps to figure out how to make movement more fun for *you*, perhaps by creating an upbeat playlist or inviting a group of your friends to go on a hike or walk together.

Day 3: Get a short burst of activity before eating A 2014 study from New Zealand found that engaging in six intense one-minute bouts of either walking on an incline, followed by one minute of slow walking, or alternating bouts of intense walking, slow walking, and bouts of resistance exercises thirty minutes before a meal helps improve blood sugar control among those with insulin resistance; the researchers dubbed this protocol "exercise snacking." My advice is to try doing this short, intense exercise approach before dinner a few times a week, in addition to your regular exercise program; you can also incorporate this approach on your "rest" days.

Day 4: Get strong during your downtime During your favorite TV show (or the commercials) or even during a phone call with a friend, do a series of squats, lunges, bicep curls, triceps dips, and front and side planks to build muscle mass and strength and tone your muscles. Instead of sitting around and reading a book, read while you pedal on a stationary bicycle or walk on a treadmill. Every little bit of movement and strength training counts!

Day 5: Set up your workout schedule Scheduling your workouts on your calendar or day-planner as if they are important medical or business appointments will make you more likely to treat that time as sacred and actually do the workouts. Take a few minutes today to schedule aerobic workouts, strength-training sessions, and other physical activities for the next thirty days—and vow to honor those health-promoting appointments.

Day 6: Start tracking Buy a pedometer or a step tracker (or track your activity on your smartphone) and aim for ten thousand steps a day, in addition to your structured exercise plan. You can do this by walking on errands, parking farther away from store entrances, and using the stairs instead of elevators. Once you launch this step, it's a keeper—something to do *every* day!

Day 7: Stretch yourself out After doing something physical, spend a few minutes stretching your major muscle groups from head to toe, to enhance your range of motion and reduce postexercise muscle soreness. This way, you'll be ready, willing, and able to stay with your exercise program. Flexibility is often the forgotten fitness factor but it can affect how you feel, move, and function in everyday life. The Cleveland Clinic's website (http://www.clevelandclinicwellness.com) provides good guides to performing basic stretches, or you could consult the book *Full-Body Flexibility* by Jay Blahnik.

Week 2: Detoxify and Rearrange Your Home

A "pure" liver starts with a clean environment and a clean diet. This week will focus on eliminating toxins from household cleaning products, as well as foods, in your home and adding more liver-friendly options.

Day 1: Pardon the pantry Clean up your pantry by eliminating processed foods (such as boxed mac and cheese, crackers made with white refined flour, junky snack foods, and anything loaded with sugar). Throw out anything that has liver no-no's (any type of sugar or syrup, or saturated fats except coconut oil) in its first five ingredients; that isn't 100 percent whole grain; that has been significantly altered from its natural state (such as reduced-fat peanut butter, butter spray, fat-free salad dressing, or anything with artificial sweeteners); and snacks that don't contain natural fiber.

Day 2: Revamp the refrigerator You don't have to go 100 percent organic with your food shopping. My advice is to use the Environmental Working Group's shopper's guides to pesticides in produce—the "Dirty Dozen" and the "Clean Fifteen" (http://www.ewg.org)—to decide which items are worth paying the extra price for the organic version. I also recommend buying organic dairy products to avoid consuming unnecessary hormones, as well as organic poultry and organic, grass-fed beef to reduce the risk of exposure to antibiotics, hormones, and bacteria.

Put the healthiest foods front and center in your fridge. For example, having a pitcher with fresh water as well as berries, cucumber,

ENVIRONMENTAL WORKING GROUP'S "DIRTY DOZEN" AND "CLEAN FIFTEEN"

Dirty Dozen	Clean Fifteen
• Strawberries	• Avocados
• Apples	• Sweet corn
• Nectarines	• Pineapples
• Peaches	• Cabbage
• Celery	• Sweet peas, frozen
• Grapes	• Onions
• Cherries	• Asparagus
• Spinach	• Mangoes
• Tomatoes	• Papayas
• Sweet bell peppers	• Kiwis
• Cherry tomatoes	• Eggplants
• Cucumbers	• Honeydew melon
• + Hot peppers	• Grapefruit
• + Kale and collard greens	• Cantaloupe
	• Cauliflower

www.ewg.org

citrus wedges, or mint on the top shelf is a great way to remind yourself to quench your thirst and walk away from food if you're not truly hungry. I'm also a fan of carbonated beverages that have flavor without artificial sweeteners. Make snacking simple by having fresh cut-up veggies (carrots, peppers, celery, and the like) available at your fingertips, near a container of hummus or almond butter. Other good options to keep on eye-level shelves include hard-boiled eggs, sticks of string cheese, and a bowl of mixed berries.

Day 3: Clean up your supplies Go through your household cleaning products and get rid of those that are loaded with toxic chemicals (if the label contains the words DANGER, WARNING, or CAUTION, that's a tip-off). Replace these with organic or naturally derived cleaning solutions (hint: the fewer ingredients and the fewer ingredients you can't pronounce on the label, the better); solutions that are water-based are generally less harmful. Also, replace plastic water bottles and food-storage containers—which often contain the chemical compound bisphenol A (BPA)—with glass or ceramic ones.

Day 4: Go wild! Whenever possible, choose wild salmon, rainbow trout, catfish, and other wild-caught fish because some farmed fish are contaminated with toxic chemicals called PCBs (polychlorinated biphenyls). To avoid another common environmental contaminant, select low-mercury fish, such as anchovies, hake, perch, pollock, salmon, sardines, shrimp, sole, tilapia, and trout; for a more complete list, check out the Natural Resources Defense Council's "Consumer Guide to Mercury in Fish": http://www.nrdc.org/health/effects/mercury/guide.asp.

Day 5: Swap your supplements Go through your medicine cabinet or kitchen cupboard, or wherever you happen to store nutritional supplements, and toss the ones that have been found to cause liver damage. These include kava, ephedra, shark cartilage, skullcap, chaparral, yohimbe, and pennyroyal, alone or in combination with other ingredients. Also, check the expiration dates on all supplement bottles, and throw away any that have passed their prime.

Day 6: Go small Start using salad or dessert plates instead of dinner plates for meals, and you'll naturally trim your portions even if you end up going back for second helpings. It also helps to keep a few everyday objects handy as useful references for how big a proper portion of meat, fish, hummus, cheese, or oil should be.

REMEMBER: 1 (3-ounce) serving of meat or chicken =
a deck of cards

1 (3-ounce) serving of fish = a checkbook

1 ounce of nuts = a golf ball

1 ounce of cheese = 3 dice

1 tablespoon of oil or hummus = a poker chip

Day 7: Embrace the season Stock your kitchen with fresh herbs, roots, and vegetables that tend to be seasonal. In the winter, look for butternut squash, sweet potatoes, and turnips; in the spring, stock up on artichokes, asparagus, basil, fiddlehead ferns, ramps, and thyme; in the summer, go for fresh corn, okra, fennel, and zucchini; and in the fall, acorn squash, Brussels sprouts, kale, lemongrass, and Swiss chard.

Week 3: Fall in Love with Your Bed Again

Sleep is when your body recharges, your cells renew themselves, and new knowledge is consolidated into memory. Neglect to give your body and mind the R & R they need, and you'll end up (literally!) throwing your body into a state of stress by triggering the release of stress hormones. This week, focus on getting back in touch with your bed.

Day 1: Set bedtime rules with your family Figure out how much sleep everyone in your family needs then set bedtimes and wake-up times accordingly. For thirty to sixty minutes before it's time to turn in, establish relaxing bedtime routines—perhaps including taking a leisurely bath, playing calming music, reading books, and the like—for your kids and for yourself. Keep bedtimes and routines consistent to set the stage for better sleep for every member of your family, night after night. If pets frequently awaken you during the night, train them to sleep in their own bed or in a crate, rather than with you; if that doesn't help sufficiently, consider banishing your pets from the bedroom.

Day 2: Create a soporific bed To enhance the quality of your nightlife, it's smart to take steps to make your bedroom a dreamy environment. Evaluate your mattress to see how comfortable and supportive it is; you should wake up feeling refreshed and well rested, not stiff or achy (if you do, it may be time to invest in a new mattress; most have a life span of about eight years, according to the National Sleep Foundation [NSF]). Whether you prefer soft or firm pillows is up to you, but they should be replaced when they lose their shape or become lumpy.

Choose sheets that feel good to you, whether they're made from a type of cotton, polyester, silk, linen, bamboo, a blend, or flannel for winter; similarly, pick a wool, cotton, or fleece blanket, depending on what suits you.

Day 3: Dim the lights Warning: Bright lights can interfere with your body's release of melatonin. A 2011 study from Brigham and Women's Hospital in Boston found that when people were exposed to standard room light before bedtime, the release of melatonin in their bodies was shortened by about ninety minutes, compared to when they spent time in a dimly lit room. That's why it's smart to do a lighting assessment to make sure your bedroom isn't too bright; once it's time to hit the sack, your bedroom should be as close to pitch black as possible. To make that happen, put dimmers on your lamps and set them to lower levels of light a few hours before bedtime. Remove all light-producing technology from your bedroom; if your alarm clock is bright, place it across the room from your bed and turn it away from you or consider swapping it for a clock that simulates light from the morning sun when it's time to get up. If streetlights or lights from nearby buildings or homes creep into your bedroom, consider installing blackout shades to eliminate unwanted light. If your bathroom is attached to your bedroom, keep the door closed, and use a motion-activated nightlight to provide you with enough light to see where you're going and what you're doing.

Day 4: Manage the temperature This day will be about finding the right bedroom temperature for you—one that's not too hot and not too cold—and the optimal clothing for snoozing. Many people find that keeping their bedroom cool—around 65°F—sets the stage for their best sleep, according to the NSF. Choose pajamas or other sleepwear that's made from a fabric that feels good against *your* skin, whether it's cotton, silk, satin, or bamboo (which is hypoallergenic). In the colder months, flannel PJs can help you stay warm while you snooze; if you tend to get hot or have night sweats while you sleep, moisture-wicking sleepwear may be your best bet because it will draw moisture away from your skin.

Day 5: Eliminate distractions Using your cell phone, tablet, e-reader, or even a TV too close to bedtime can leave you counting sheep when it's time to turn in. The reason: The light emitted by these devices may suppress your body's release of sleep-inducing melatonin. The solution is to impose a no-technology rule at least one to two hours before bedtime; that means no e-mails, no television, no e-readers, laptops or mobile phones. Instead, opt for a relaxing activity that will help you downshift from your workday and put you in the mood to snooze. If cutting yourself off from technology one to two hours before bedtime seems impossible, at least banish technology from the bedroom in the evenings.

Day 6: Get a grip on stimulants Identify stimulants in your evening routine and eliminate them. Remember: Drinking tea or coffee or eating chocolate or coffee-flavored ice cream or yogurt in the evening could interfere with your slumber, so it's best to avoid these foods and beverages for four to six hours before bedtime. Similarly, nicotine in cigarettes has a stimulating effect so steer clear of smoking (which you should be doing anyway) in the evening, at the very least. Also, keep in mind that while alcohol can make you feel sleepy initially, it can have a stimulating effect a few hours later, leading to fragmented sleep—another good reason to keep your intake to a minimum. On the other hand, remember that some sleep aids—such as Tylenol PM—contain acetaminophen along with diphenhydramine (a sedating antihistamine); in large doses, acetaminophen is toxic to the liver, especially when it's combined with alcohol, and this is true whether you take a daytime formula or a nighttime one.

Day 7: Indulge yourself To set the stage for better sleep, establish nighttime rituals that feel good and quiet your mind. These could include taking a warm bath, stretching or doing yoga, listening to soothing music, using aromatherapy, breathing deeply or meditating, and/or reading an enjoyable book that isn't too stimulating. Engaging in activities that relax your mind and body will help you make the journey to dreamland more easily.

Week 4: Find Your Decompression Valve

It's not the stress in your life that makes you sick, irritable, or exhausted—it's your response to it! During week 4, you'll gain the tools you need to recognize and manage your stress better from now on. (Using the "Stress-Trigger Tracking Sheet," found in Appendix C, can help in this respect.)

Day 1: Get in touch with your breath We're born knowing how to breathe, but believe it or not, many people don't breathe properly (they breathe too shallowly). Breathing deeply is one of the most powerful antidotes to feeling stressed: When you inhale slowly and deeply through your nose, letting air fill your lungs as your lower belly expands, then exhale slowly through your mouth, you'll get the proper exchange of oxygen for outgoing carbon dioxide; this exchange will slow your heartbeat and blood pressure and induce the relaxation response, a state of profound calm. Take a five- to ten-minute break two or three times per day to check in with how you're breathing and make a point to engage in deep breathing. It will allow you to better manage your stress and help it dissipate.

Day 2: Take meditation breaks Meditation can provide a powerful source of calmness and stress relief—anytime, anywhere, and for no cost at all. Just ask Krista, a 46-year-old stay-at-home mother with two kids, who had been coming to see me for six months with the goal of losing 15 pounds, the last remnants of her "baby weight." Although she was reluctant to admit it, life was stressful for her: Besides having two young kids, her ailing mother was living with the family and Krista's husband traveled on business four to five days a week. Krista had cut calories, but she often ate for emotional reasons (usually sweets) and constantly made excuses about never having the time or energy to exercise. Some of her reasons were legitimate, but at least three days a week, she had a nanny to look after her kids, and she had a fairly extensive gym in her home.

Since stress management was clearly a challenge for her, she finally agreed to see a mindfulness expert for *one* session. After that, Krista began meditating three times a day, as well as doing breathing exercises and guided imagery exercises. Within a few months, she started exercising again, and her eating habits and portion control improved, as well. When I asked her what made the difference, she credited her meditation practice with helping her to become more open to the steps she needed to take to shed the excess weight. In hindsight, she realized that she'd been operating on autopilot, which created weight-management challenges she hadn't even been aware of.

Here is an easy meditation technique. To reap the benefits, practice two to three times a day to help you stay centered, calm, and focused.

1. Find a quiet, peaceful place—a room or simply a corner of a room—where you can be alone.

2. Sit on a straight-backed chair or cross-legged on the floor, with your back straight, your hands on your knees or thighs, and your eyes closed.

3. To begin clearing your mind through basic mindfulness meditation, focus on the natural rhythm of your breathing; when thoughts come to mind, allow them to simply pass without judging or engaging them, as if they were leaves floating on a stream, and return your attention to your breathing.

Day 3: Take a walk in nature In addition to your usual exercise plan, taking short walks in green areas—such as a park, the woods, or along a trail—can help soothe stress. To maximize the experience, it helps to engage your senses: look at the flowers, foliage, wildlife, or views around you; remove your earbuds and listen to the birds chirping or the wind rustling through the trees; smell the roses, lilacs, or honeysuckle as you pass by; and enjoy the warmth of the sun or the coolness of the breeze on your skin. Spending time in nature can take your mind away from your everyday worries and bring it to a place of tranquility. Even if it's cold outside, take a walk around the block and appreciate the light and the winter landscape.

Day 4: Use your imagination for a midday vacation Harnessing the power of guided imagery to steer your mind to a calmer place can help you relax quickly. Try this ten-minute exercise:

1. Find a comfy chair in a quiet space and sit in a position that feels good to you.

2. Close your eyes, breathe slowly and deeply, and picture the most relaxing place you can imagine, whether it's the calm, clear ocean near a tropical island or a spectacular vista at the top of a mountain.

3. As you visualize this relaxing scene, try to recruit all your senses to imagine what the place looks like, what sounds you'd hear, what smells you'd experience, and how the air would feel against your skin. Bask in those sensations and let yourself drift away from reality, in a well-deserved mental mini-vacation.

Day 5: Create a stress-relieving toolkit Make a list of reliable strategies that help you tame your tension—perhaps writing in a journal, listening to soothing music, calling an old friend, doing progressive muscle relaxation exercises, and the like. Post it on your fridge so you can turn to one of these healthy strategies rather than eating for emotional reasons the next time your stress meter registers overload.

Day 6: Identify a fulfilling hobby you enjoy It could be knitting, drawing, taking photographs, cooking, or doing something else altogether. Getting your mind engaged in an engrossing activity that's truly appealing to you can help you achieve "flow"—a mental state in which you're so fully immersed and focused on what you're doing that you lose track of time passing, which naturally has a stress-relieving effect. What's more, activities that put you in that optimal zone tend to be intrinsically rewarding and lead to feelings of serenity and satisfaction. Pinpoint activities that have this sort of effect on you, and make an effort to carve out time on a regular basis to engage in them.

Day 7: Identify your go-to person Knowing that you have a reliable, unconditionally supportive person you can turn to when you're in a jam or feeling wretched or you need advice on how to continue with the healthy lifestyle changes you're trying to make can help you manage stress better and make strides toward your health-related goals. It's best to seek someone who has your optimal interests in mind and can serve as your cheerleader, motivate you to stay on course, and keep you accountable for your actions. If the person actually shares your goal of getting healthier, that may be the most ideal scenario of all. Sometimes even a cyber buddy can spur you on to great achievements. A 2012 study from Michigan State University found that having a virtually present partner helped participants hold plank exercises longer and work harder than those who undertook the challenge on their own. This means that if you're struggling to find someone to hold your hand through challenges, you can always enlist the help of an online coach or someone from your social media network.

Taking steps to upgrade your lifestyle habits in a week-by-week, day-by-day fashion will make the undertaking much less daunting and much more manageable. The goal is to build upon the strategies you implemented the day before so that you continue to make changes in an upward, synergistic pattern that will provide built-in positive reinforcement. Keep up the good work every day and before you know it, you'll have developed healthy habits that will enhance the state of your liver and the rest of your body, as well as your mind. Ultimately, this will translate into better overall health, a boost in your energy, and fortified resolve that will help you stick with your feel-good liver-protection plan for the long haul.

chapter 12

Other Treatments

A FEW YEARS AGO, Jim, 59, a computer engineer, came to the Cleveland Clinic's liver clinic for evaluation because he was experiencing abdominal discomfort. For many years, he'd had abnormal liver enzyme levels and a body mass index (BMI) of 45, which is considered morbidly obese, a state that led to his developing fatty liver disease in the first place. An abdominal ultrasound revealed that Jim's liver had a coarse texture that's consistent with liver cirrhosis. Fortunately, he didn't have complications from liver cirrhosis such as ascites (an accumulation of fluid in the abdomen), gastrointestinal bleeding, or mental confusion due to an accumulation of toxins in the body (a condition called hepatic encephalopathy).

At that point, his liver seemed to be compensating reasonably well for the damage it had suffered and it was still functioning well enough. But if Jim didn't take dramatic steps to reverse the damage, it would have worsened, setting him up for possible liver failure and/ or the prospect of needing a liver transplant. Fortunately, the married father of two was motivated to improve his health because he wanted to live long enough to play with his grandkids. To jump-start the process, Jim chose to undergo gastric bypass surgery and he lost 45 pounds over a three-month period after the surgery.

Thanks to his significant weight loss, Jim's previously elevated blood pressure returned to normal and he was able to stop taking the hypertension medicine he'd been taking before the surgery. At the six-month and one-year milestones after the surgery, Jim returned to the liver clinic for follow-up evaluations and his liver enzyme levels were normal both times. At his two-year follow-up visit, he had a liver biopsy performed, which showed that the cirrhosis had regressed to a milder state of stage 3 fibrosis—still a cause for concern but a major step in the right direction.

By and large, the treatment for nonalcoholic fatty liver disease (NAFLD) doesn't usually involve medications or surgery. As you've seen, it is based primarily on modifying your lifestyle habits by improving your diet, exercising more, and losing excess weight. But if lifestyle measures alone don't help sufficiently with weight reduction and fat loss from the liver, stronger measures may be in order, as they were for Jim.

Medication Matters

The reality is that specific medications haven't been approved for the treatment of NAFLD or nonalcoholic steatohepatitis (NASH). But for severe cases of NASH that don't respond sufficiently to lifestyle changes or weight loss, medications can be beneficial in some instances.

Insulin-sensitizing agents and lipid-lowering agents For starters, insulin-sensitizing agents and lipid-lowering agents may benefit the liver of people who have NAFLD as well as diabetes or cholesterol abnormalities. As you've learned, insulin resistance and metabolic syndrome are commonly associated with NAFLD and NASH, so it makes sense that insulin-sensitizing drugs, such as metformin, pioglitazone, and rosiglitazone, might help. A 2005 study from Italy compared the effects of giving nondiabetic patients with NAFLD 2 grams of metformin or 800 IU of vitamin E daily or a weight-reduction diet: After twelve months, aspartate aminotransferase (AST) levels improved in all three groups, in conjunction with weight loss, but the effects were greatest in the metformin group, of which 56 percent also experienced normalization of their alanine aminotransferase (ALT) levels; a subset of patients receiving metformin had liver biopsies and were found to have a significant decrease in liver fat and fibrosis. Since most nondiabetic patients with NASH have glucose intolerance (or insulin resistance), metformin has the added benefit of lowering their risk of developing full-blown diabetes. Other studies, however, haven't found a significant benefit from giving metformin to people with NAFLD or NASH, so the effects aren't guaranteed to be a sure thing.

There has been considerable interest in another class of insulin-sensitizing agents called thiazolidinediones, which includes the drugs pioglitazone and rosiglitazone, for the treatment of NASH. As with metformin, these drugs sensitize the liver to insulin and reduce liver enzyme levels. The thiazolidinediones seem to have a more favorable effect on the infiltration of fat in the liver (steatosis) than on inflammation, ballooning, or fibrosis. Unfortunately, their beneficial effects on the liver grind to a halt when the drugs are discontinued, which suggests that long-term treatment is required to maintain the therapeutic effects. This is of concern because there have been questions about the long-term safety of rosiglitazone, in particular, when it comes to cardiovascular disease, congestive heart failure, bladder cancer, and bone loss; due to the increased risk of heart problems, rosiglitazone is no longer sold in Europe and it is used on a highly restrictive basis in the United States.

Recently, liraglutide, another drug that's used to treat type 2 diabetes, was found to be beneficial in the management of NASH. In theory, this long-acting drug should reduce fat on the liver and decrease liver enzyme levels by improving insulin resistance—and there's some evidence that this may be true. A 2015 study conducted in several different locations in the United Kingdom found that when overweight patients with NASH were given 1.8 mg of liraglutide daily (as injections) for forty-eight weeks, 39 percent of them experienced resolution of their NASH, compared to 9 percent of those who were given a placebo. Similarly, in a small 2015 pilot study, researchers from Japan gave liraglutide to people whose blood sugar levels and/or ALT liver enzyme levels hadn't improved enough with lifestyle modifications after twenty-four weeks; after getting liraglutide for an additional twenty-four weeks, the patients experienced significant improvements in their BMI, abdominal fat levels, liver enzyme levels, and blood sugar abnormalities. In both studies, the treatment was well tolerated, safe, and effective. More research needs to be done before this drug becomes widely used but so far the results are encouraging.

Statins In a completely different line of attack, several small, preliminary studies have suggested that statins, used primarily to treat cholesterol abnormalities, may reduce elevated liver enzymes and improve the appearance of liver tissue (when viewed under a microscope) in people with NAFLD or NASH. A 2011 study from Japan found that when patients with NASH who also had cholesterol abnormalities were given statin drugs daily, their liver enzyme levels and lipid profiles improved significantly after a year. More recently, a 2014 study from Hiroshima University in Japan investigated the use of an older anticholesterol drug called probucol, which is a powerful antioxidant, in people who have NASH and elevated cholesterol levels: After taking 500 mg of the drug daily for forty-eight weeks, their liver enzyme levels, total cholesterol levels, and insulin resistance indexes decreased, and their NAFLD scores and stages of fibrosis improved as well.

Antioxidants

Since excessive oxidative stress (an imbalance between the production of damaging free radicals and the body's ability to counteract or neutralize their effects) can lead to injury of liver cells and disease progression in people with NASH, it's not surprising that some potent antioxidants could be beneficial in the treatment of NASH.

Vitamin E In the largest clinical trial yet, the results of which were published in a 2010 issue of the *New England Journal of Medicine*, researchers found that giving adults with NASH 800 IU of vitamin E daily for ninety-six weeks led to a significantly higher rate of improvement in their condition than a placebo did, including reductions in fat content on the liver, inflammation, and elevated liver enzymes. One of the biggest concerns with vitamin E supplements is that taking high doses may be associated with an increased risk of premature mortality from any cause, though the research on this subject has yielded mixed results. Nevertheless, because vitamin E supplementation has been found to be so effective in reducing fat, inflammation, and ballooning in the liver, and even resolving NASH in some patients who have it, vitamin E (800 IU daily) should be considered as a first-line form of pharmacotherapy for nondiabetic patients with NASH that's been confirmed by biopsy.

This was the case for Paul, 55, who had been referred to Dr. Ha-nouneh because he was suspected to have fatty liver disease. His health had been steady until about three months earlier when he be-gan getting headaches and went to see his primary care physician. A respiratory therapist who is married and has two young children, Paul was found to have hypertension, a BMI of 38, and significant abdominal obesity. A battery of initial blood tests revealed that his fasting blood sugar was normal, his triglycerides were moderately elevated at 220 mg/dl, and his HDL (the "good") cholesterol was low at 25 mg/dl. Follow-up blood tests indicated his liver enzymes were elevated—his AST was 110 (the upper limit of normal is 40), and his ALT was 145 (the upper limit is 56). His alcohol intake was light to moderate and the results of his screening tests for hepatitis B and C were negative. An ultrasound of his liver showed fatty liver, so Paul had a liver biopsy, which showed that 35 percent of the liver tissue that normally removes toxins was occupied by fat, along with inflam-mation and stage 1 fibrosis.

Paul was advised to lose weight by modifying his diet and exercis-ing through a strict weight-loss program. Because there was a sense of urgency to stopping the damage to his liver, he was started on a protocol of 800 IU of vitamin E daily to support his liver while he was losing weight. He was counseled that large doses of vitamin E might be associated with an increased risk of heart attack or stroke and an increased risk of prostate cancer. After a year on the weight-loss pro-gram, he lost 25 pounds, which resulted in complete normalization of his liver enzyme levels; at that point, he stopped taking vitamin E to avoid the risks of long-term adverse effects.

Coenzyme Q10 Another powerful antioxidant, coenzyme Q10 (a.k.a. ubiquinone) is a vitamin-like substance that's found in our cells and assists in the process of converting food into usable forms of energy. It also may play a role in reversing the severity of NAFLD. In a 2015 study from Iran, researchers gave forty-one men and women with NA-FLD 100 mg of coenzyme Q10 daily for twelve weeks; at the end of the study, their liver enzyme levels improved, their measures of inflam-mation went down, and the severity of their NAFLD decreased, as well. Another study from Iran found that taking 100 mg of coenzyme

Q10 for just four weeks led to a significant decrease in AST levels, among patients with NAFLD.

New drugs Meanwhile, the development of pharmacological treatments for severe NAFLD are gaining traction, and the Food and Drug Administration has granted fast-track status to a new program designed to expedite the review of new drugs that are being developed to treat NAFLD and NASH. Already, several recent studies have found that pentoxifylline, an anti-inflammatory agent, leads to weight loss, improved liver function, as well as reduced fat accumulation and inflammation in people with NASH. And a recent study found that a medication called obeticholic acid, a bile acid signaler, improves NASH in many cases, but the long-term benefits and safety profile need further investigation. With more studies under way, new treatments for these potentially life-threatening diseases will hopefully emerge.

Bariatric Surgery

When lifestyle modifications, weight loss, and/or medications can't reverse the damage from NASH, bariatric surgery may be an option for some people, as it was in Jim's case. While there aren't any randomized controlled trials that have evaluated any form of foregut bariatric surgery—such as adjustable gastric banding and Roux-en-Y gastric bypass—to specifically treat NAFLD or NASH, there is mounting evidence of its effectiveness in this context. Several studies have done a before-and-after comparison of the liver in severely obese people who had bariatric surgery: In a 2009 study, researchers from France examined the effects of bariatric surgery in 381 severely obese patients who had fibrosis and NASH. Five years after the surgery, there was a significant improvement in the prevalence and severity of fat content and ballooning in the liver and the vast majority of the patients had their conditions downgraded to low levels of NAFLD. Meanwhile, a 2015 study from France found that when morbidly obese people with NASH underwent bariatric surgery, they lost significant amounts of weight and gained major improvements

OTHER LIVER DISEASES, OTHER INTERVENTIONS

Just as the causes of various liver diseases vary, the treatments do, too. Hepatitis C now can be treated and cured in as little as eight to twelve weeks, thanks to five different drugs that are now approved for use in the United States (warning: many of the drugs are very expensive). The treatment for alcohol-related liver disease, including alcoholic hepatitis and alcoholic fatty liver disease (AFLD), focuses on abstaining from alcohol and allowing the liver to regenerate and heal itself. When it comes to primary biliary cholangitis (PBC), treatment is aimed at slowing the progression of the disease, alleviating symptoms (such as itching), and preventing complications with the use of such medications as ursodiol (to improve the liver's ability to function).

By contrast, treatment for hemochromatosis (a genetic condition involving iron overload) involves reducing the amount of iron that has accumulated in the liver; this is often done through phlebotomy (removing a small amount of iron-laden blood in a procedure similar to blood donation) or chelation therapy (which relies on a medication that causes your body to expel iron through your urine or stool). Similarly, treatment for Wilson disease uses various methods (including such drugs as penicillamine, trientine, and zinc acetate) to eliminate excess copper from the body.

in their liver enzyme levels and their insulin resistance; at the one-year follow-up, NASH had disappeared entirely from 85 percent of the patients and fibrosis was reduced in 34 percent of the patients.

The Truth about Transplants

It's important to remember that the liver is a remarkably resilient organ, one that's capable of rebuilding and regenerating itself using its own cells to replace the tissue that was lost to disease—until it returns to its original size. But with some liver diseases, this vital organ can become so damaged that it reaches a point of no return—that's when someone becomes a candidate for a liver transplant.

By itself, cirrhosis doesn't necessarily imply a need for a liver transplant; some patients who have liver cirrhosis without complications don't experience a complete breakdown in function or a full decay of the liver. In fact, with many types of liver disease, there's the potential for improvement even after complications have occurred—if an alcoholic patient experiences liver decay, complete with jaundice and other signs of advanced liver disease, he or she may experience a resolution of these symptoms and regeneration of the liver with long-term abstinence from alcohol. So, in some cases where patients have marked liver deterioration, the prospect of a liver transplant may be deferred or even shelved entirely if medical therapies (such as oral antiviral agents for hepatitis B infection or corticosteroid drugs for autoimmune hepatitis) are effective.

But when cirrhosis and the complications that often come with it reach a certain point, as in end-stage liver disease, it's time to have a serious discussion with your doctor about the possibility of having a liver transplant. When NAFLD and NASH progress to the point of cirrhosis of the liver with such complications as ascites, hepatic encephalopathy, variceal hemorrhage (rupturing and bleeding from swollen veins), or severe liver dysfunction, transplantation may be considered. The good news is the one-year survival rate after a liver transplant is higher than 90 percent and the five-year survival rate is more than 70 percent. These figures are outstanding, especially compared to the nearly 100 percent mortality rate that's associated with end-stage liver disease that isn't treated with a liver transplant.

After a liver transplant, patients need to take antirejection medicines for the rest of their life. Unfortunately, these drugs are not without side effects. Tacrolimus, the most commonly used antirejection medicine, is associated with kidney toxicity, so renal function should be monitored closely in patients who take the drug. Moreover, the drug is also linked with an increased risk of a new onset of diabetes after a liver transplant, so blood sugar should be monitored closely, too. By contrast, the use of cyclosporine, another commonly used antirejection drug, is associated with an increased risk of hypertension following a liver transplant.

Since antirejection drugs lead to immunosuppression, they increase the risk of infectious complications after a liver transplant, so it's not unusual for transplant recipients to be given prophylactic antibiotics, such as Bactrim, for the rest of their life. But this doesn't protect them from other infections—from viruses or fungi, for example—so it's important to remember that this increased vulnerability persists, which is why transplant patients should get an annual flu vaccine and the pneumonia vaccine. Because of these potential long-term risks, all liver transplant patients need to be monitored closely and regularly by their liver transplant team for the rest of their life.

It's important to recognize, too, that there's often a long waiting list for a liver transplant, so not everyone who needs one will get one in time. What's more, not everyone with complications due to liver cirrhosis is a good candidate for a transplant. In those who are morbidly obese or have severe complications related to diabetes or heart disease, having a liver transplant may be too risky to be a viable option. This is something that only your physician can determine. But ideally you want to prevent that triple- (or quadruple-) threat scenario from occurring in the first place.

While it's comforting to know that more aggressive and effective treatments are being developed for NAFLD, NASH, and other liver disorders, it's best to do whatever you can to protect the health and integrity of this vital organ now, long before the liver turns down the path to serious degeneration. Even if you already have one of these liver disorders, you can take steps to set the wheel of disease-reversal into motion (or at least stop its progression) and improve the health of this crucial organ. So, it's essential to be proactive! Given our collective lifestyle that promotes the development of obesity, we're all potentially at risk for NAFLD, and NASH in particular, which means we should all make an effort to improve our diet and exercise habits, manage our weight more effectively, and avoid toxic exposures. It could be a matter of life or death, because our entire body really does depend on the health, well-being, and functionality of this indispensable organ.

Liver for Life

Is life worth living? It all depends on the liver.
—AMERICAN PSYCHOLOGIST AND PHILOSOPHER
WILLIAM JAMES

Our hope is that by now you've gained a newfound respect for your liver, one of the hardest-working organs in your body. Our hope is that after reading this book you'll be motivated to give this crucial organ the proper care and feeding it needs and deserves to stay healthy and thrive—and keep you healthy and thriving for life. As you've seen, this magician-like organ is the silent but powerful master behind the curtain, playing a vital and invaluable role in your body's ability to perform more than three hundred tasks, involving metabolic processes, detoxifying effects, digestive functions, and more. And yet, even though it's on duty 24/7, it's largely forgotten in the noise and chaos of daily life.

To some extent it's human nature to take for granted what we can't see, sense, or feel—and that tendency may play a role in why we don't pay enough attention to the liver. But the truth is that you rely on your liver, and knowingly or not, you expect a lot from it because as you've seen, your liver is essential to your health, well-being, and survival; however, it can't perform its myriad jobs without your help. If you abuse your liver by packing on too much body fat, consuming a junk-food diet, maintaining a couch potato mentality, drinking too much alcohol, or engaging in other unhealthy lifestyle habits—you can develop a fatty, low-grade liver. Picture it as an ugly, marbled, grizzled, or even rotting piece of meat: You wouldn't buy a steak that looked like that at the grocery store or accept it at a fancy restaurant—so why on earth would you risk letting an indispensable part of your own body grow to look that way? *Don't!*

It's time for all of us to give our liver the care and respect it needs and deserves—before problems develop. As you've seen, the proactive approach outlined in this book doesn't have to be as complicated as you may have feared. Start by focusing on low-hanging fruit—easy, everyday tweaks you can make to your habits—and build from there. First, add as much color as you can from Mother Nature's garden (fruits, vegetables, nuts, and seeds). Then, swap refined grains for whole grains and bad fats for healthy ones. Trade your evening habit of winding down with a glass of wine (or two) for a steaming mug (or two) of decaffeinated tea. Start moving more: You don't need to run a marathon; just strive to do more physical activity today than you did yesterday, and each day, aim for another step, another minute, another breathless moment of exertion and you'll do your body a world of good. But also take time to breathe—deeply!—and decompress regularly so that your psychological stress doesn't lead to stress for your liver.

On a weekly basis, we see people who have revamped their habits, reduced toxins in their environments, gained a grip on life-threatening health conditions, such as nonalcoholic steatohepatitis (NASH), and turned their health prognoses around in the process. We see how much they value the improvements that are evident in the results of their blood work, on the scale, and in the way they feel and function. You, too, have the power and the wherewithal to alter your lifestyle in ways that will safeguard your liver and help it to perform its essential jobs in an optimal fashion, just as have many of the patients described in this book.

Whether the measures that are most pertinent to you involve improving the quality of your diet, becoming more physically active, shedding excess weight, quitting smoking, and/or reducing your exposure to harmful chemicals, these health-promoting changes will have positive ripple effects on all your other organs. That's right—they'll benefit your heart, lungs, digestive system, brain, and the rest of you, not only because these lifestyle modifications will have a directly positive influence on these other organ systems, but also because the state of your liver can affect how well your brain, heart, lungs, digestive tract, and kidneys function. You really can create a positive cascade of health perks for your entire body and mind. In addition, these lifestyle upgrades will improve your energy and your overall sense of well-being, and they will help protect your long-term health, vitality, and longevity.

When it comes right down to it, this really is a no-lose proposition! You're the only one who can make this happen—and we urge you to do just that. Think of this liver-protection plan as your free ticket to a longer, more energized and vibrant life. It's yours for the taking. Think of it as an investment in extending the quality of your life well into the future. If you think of your liver as the guardian angel of your health, you'll be more likely to do whatever you can to protect its halo and help this vital organ help you stay healthy. Indeed, by making your liver health a priority, you'll be making the rest of your health and well-being a priority, too. And this will set the stage for you to thrive in various aspects of your life, which is as it should be. We encourage you to embark on this journey to a happier, healthier you, starting today. We will be cheering you on from the sidelines!

Recipes

For clarity's sake, the recipes that follow have been flagged with an icon to indicate whether they're included in the Love-Your-Liver Eating Plan **LYL** (Chapter 9) or the Skinny Liver Diet **SL** (Chapter 10).

BREAKFAST
Green Smoothie
Energizing Kale Smoothie
Tropical Breakfast Bowl
Overnight Soaked Oats
Zucchini Muffins
Crustless Quiche Cups
Veggie Quinoa Quiche Cups

Green Smoothie **LYL**

Packed with greens and liver-protective hemp seeds and spirulina, this smoothie is a terrific way to start the day—or enjoy as a midday boost.

SERVES 4

1 cup roughly chopped, firmly packed kale
1 cup roughly chopped, firmly packed romaine lettuce
1 cup green seedless grapes
1 Bartlett pear, stemmed and cored
1 orange, peeled, pith removed, and quartered
1 banana, peeled
1 teaspoon hemp seeds
1 teaspoon spirulina

½ cup coconut water
2 cups ice

Place all the ingredients in a blender and process on low speed for 15 seconds. Increase to medium speed, then high speed. Process until well blended.

Energizing Kale Smoothie LYL

You may be accustomed to using avocado in salads and guacamole; its creamy richness pairs well with fruit and greens for a filling breakfast treat, too.

SERVES 1

1 frozen banana, chopped
½ cup plain low-fat yogurt
½ cup blueberries
1 cup packed chopped kale
½ ripe avocado
½ cup unsweetened almond milk

Place all the ingredients in a blender and process at high speed until they reach a desired consistency. Serve immediately.

Tropical Breakfast Bowl LYL

A great source of fiber, whole-grain oats can help you start the day well nourished, with satiety and staying power that can help you get through the morning. With the sweetness of mango and coconut, it's a bit of an island retreat.

SERVES 1

1 cup unsweetened almond milk
½ cup whole-grain oats
½ cup mango chunks
2 tablespoons chopped walnuts
1 tablespoon unsweetened coconut flakes

Combine the almond milk and oats in a small, microwave-safe bowl. Microwave on HIGH for 6 minutes. Stir, then let it stand for 2 minutes. Top with the mango chunks, walnuts, and coconut flakes.

Overnight Soaked Oats LYL

If you find yourself running out of time in the morning and missing breakfast, this simple dish is for you. For an even easier grab-and-go approach, mix all the ingredients in a jar and just put the jar in your bag on your way out the door.

SERVES 1

½ cup old-fashioned rolled oats
1 cup unsweetened almond milk
2 tablespoons almond butter
1 tablespoon honey

Mix all the ingredients together well in a medium-size bowl. Cover and store in the fridge. Enjoy cold or heat in a microwave the next morning.

Zucchini Muffins LYL

Whip up a batch of these on the weekend and freeze half in individual bags for a healthy alternative to your morning pastry.

MAKES 12 MUFFINS

Coconut oil cooking spray
1 cup walnuts or pecans
2 cups blanched almond flour
1 teaspoon ground allspice
1 teaspoon ground nutmeg
1 teaspoon ground cinnamon
1 ¼ teaspoons baking soda
½ teaspoon sea salt
1 teaspoon pure vanilla extract

2 large or 3 medium zucchini, grated
4 large eggs
⅓ cup applesauce
¼ cup extra-virgin coconut oil, melted

Preheat the oven to 350°F. Grease a twelve-cup muffin pan with coconut oil cooking spray.

Grind the walnuts or pecans in a food processor until coarse. Combine the ground nuts, almond flour, spices, baking soda, and salt in a small bowl.

Meanwhile, mix the vanilla, grated zucchini, eggs, applesauce, and coconut oil together in a large bowl. Add the dry ingredients to the wet ingredients and stir well to combine.

Divide the mixture equally among the prepared muffin cups and bake for 30 minutes. You'll know they're done when a knife or toothpick inserted into the center of a muffin comes out clean. They can be stored in the fridge for up to 5 days.

Crustless Quiche Cups🆂🅻

Eggs have gotten a bad rap in recent years, but they are full of protein and essential vitamins and minerals. Whip them up with some veggies for this traditional breakfast favorite.

SERVES 6

Nonstick cooking spray
1 (10-ounce) package frozen chopped kale, or 2 cups chopped fresh
2 large eggs, plus 3 large egg whites
¼ cup chopped leek
¼ cup chopped sun-dried tomato
¼ cup seeded and chopped yellow bell pepper

Preheat the oven to 350°F. Line a six-cup muffin pan with paper liners and spray with nonstick cooking spray.

If using frozen kale, microwave it for 2½ minutes on HIGH, then drain away the excess liquid. Combine the eggs, egg whites, leek, sun-dried tomatoes, kale, and bell pepper in a bowl and mix well. Divide the mixture equally among the prepared muffin cups.

Bake for 20 minutes, or until a knife comes out clean after being inserted in the center.

Note: These will stay fresh in the fridge for a few days, but they don't freeze well.

Veggie Quinoa Quiche Cups🆂🄻

Quinoa is the star here; this ancient seed adds a protein boost to this cheesy, eggy dish.

SERVES 6

Nonstick cooking spray
½ cup uncooked quinoa, rinsed
2 tablespoons olive oil
1 Vidalia onion, thinly sliced
4 cups washed and torn or chopped spinach leaves
1 garlic clove, minced
½ shallot, chopped
Sea salt and freshly ground black pepper
½ cup shredded low-fat Cheddar cheese
½ cup grated Parmesan cheese
2 large eggs, plus 4 large egg whites, lightly beaten

Preheat the oven to 375°F. Line a six-cup muffin pan with paper liners and spray with nonstick cooking spray; set aside.

Combine 1 cup of water and the quinoa in a small saucepan and bring to a boil. Lower the heat to a simmer, cover, and continue to cook for 15 minutes, then remove from the heat, remove the lid, and allow the cooked quinoa to cool.

Heat the olive oil in a large skillet over medium heat, add the onion, and cook until the onion is translucent, 3 to 4 minutes. Stir in the spinach, garlic, and shallot. Season to taste with salt and pepper and continue to cook until the spinach is wilted, about 2 more minutes. Remove the pan from the heat and let the mixture cool.

Combine the cooked quinoa, the spinach mixture, and the cheeses in a large mixing bowl. Pour in the eggs and egg whites and mix well to combine the ingredients.

Divide the batter evenly among the prepared muffin cups. Bake for 35 minutes, or until the quiche tops are golden brown.

Note: These will stay fresh in the fridge for a few days, but they don't freeze well.

SALADS & SOUPS

Salads
Broccoli Salad
Seaweed Salad
Apple, Pear, and Jicama Waldorf Salad
Shaved Brussels Sprouts Salad
Mango, Avocado, and Black Bean Salad
Mango Quinoa Salad
Beet and Orange Salad
Roasted Beet Salad
Warm Mushroom and Kale Salad
Kale Pesto and Barley Salad
Kale and Apple Salad
Zucchini and Farro Salad
Dandelion Greens Salad with Sprouted Pumpkin Seeds
Blackberry Freekeh Salad
Crispy Chickpea Salad
Chicken Salad
Albacore Tuna Salad
Wild Shrimp and Black Bean Salad

Broccoli Salad ⑤

Broccoli's not the only crunch here; pistachios, carrots, and bell pepper add flavor and texture. If you find yourself with extra dressing, save it for a simple green salad.

SERVES 4

1 cup broccoli florets
¼ cup chopped red onion
1 cup shredded carrot
¼ cup seeded and chopped orange bell pepper
⅓ cup chopped pistachios
1 clementine orange, separated into segments

FOR THE DRESSING:
1 teaspoon minced fresh garlic
1 tablespoon extra-virgin olive oil
¼ cup freshly squeezed orange juice
Freshly ground black pepper

Combine the broccoli, red onion, carrot, bell pepper, pistachios, and orange segments in a large bowl.

Prepare the dressing: Whisk together the dressing ingredients in a small bowl, seasoning to taste with black pepper. Pour the dressing onto the salad and mix well. Let the salad chill for at least 1 hour to allow the flavors to combine. Serve chilled.

Seaweed Salad⑤

If you're new to sea vegetables, don't be intimidated. You'll find that seaweed pairs wonderfully with this dressing for an easy, delicious way to get protein and key nutrients into your diet.

SERVES 4

2 ounces dried mixed seaweed

FOR THE DRESSING
2 tablespoons rice vinegar
1 teaspoon coconut sugar
2 teaspoons ground ginger
½ teaspoon wasabi powder
2 teaspoons low-sodium soy sauce
1 tablespoon roasted sesame oil

Juice of 1 lime
Sea salt
1 small carrot, peeled and sliced paper thin
5 red radishes, thinly sliced
1 small cucumber, peeled and thinly sliced
2 teaspoons toasted black sesame seeds
2 teaspoons hemp seeds
4 green onions or scallions, slivered

Put the seaweed in a large bowl and cover with cold water. Let soak for 5 to 10 minutes, until softened. Drain in a colander, pat dry, and place in a serving bowl.

To make the dressing, whisk together the vinegar, coconut sugar, ginger, wasabi powder, soy sauce, and sesame oil in a small bowl.

Spoon half of the dressing over the seaweed, add the lime juice, and toss gently. Taste and add a small amount of salt if necessary.

Surround the salad with the carrot, radish, and cucumber slices. Season lightly with salt and drizzle with the remaining dressing, then sprinkle the salad with the black sesame seeds, hemp seeds, and green onions.

Apple, Pear, and Jicama Waldorf Salad 🆂🅛

I created this recipe with Chef Jim Perko; it first appeared on Dr. Oz's website. Apples and pears can help you lose weight and give you better blood sugar control. What better way to enjoy them than with liver-supporting jicama?

SERVES 10

1 pound jicama
2 cups unsweetened pineapple juice
3 Fuji apples
3 pears, in a variety of colors
2 cups red grapes
½ cup walnuts, chopped and toasted
¼ cup unsalted sunflower seeds
½ cup raisins, red or yellow
12 ounces nondairy mayonnaise
½ cup almonds, sliced and toasted

Peel the jicama, dice into small pieces, then place in a bowl with the pineapple juice to prevent browning, about 2 minutes. Drain the jicama, reserving the liquid for the other fruit.

Wash, core, and dice the apples and place them in the reserved pineapple juice to prevent browning, about 2 minutes. Drain the apples, reserving the liquid in the bowl.

Wash, core and dice the pears and place them in the pineapple juice to prevent browning. Let the pears soak in the pineapple juice while you wash and cut the grapes in half. Drain the pears, reserving the liquid in the bowl.

Combine and mix all the ingredients, including the reserved pineapple juice, in a large bowl.

Shaved Brussels Sprouts Salad ⓢⓛ

This easy recipe shows off these little cruciferous veggies in their best light: dressed simply, the bright flavors really shine.

SERVES 8

1¾ pounds Brussels sprouts, trimmed, outer leaves removed
5 tablespoons extra-virgin olive oil
12 medium-size shallots, thinly sliced (about 2 cups)
6 garlic cloves, thinly sliced
2 tablespoons freshly squeezed lemon juice
Sea salt and freshly ground black pepper

Working in small batches, place the Brussels sprouts in the feeding tube of a food processor that has been fitted with a thin slicing disk and slice the sprouts. Alternatively, slice them by hand into thin slices.

Heat the olive oil in a large pot over medium heat and sauté the shallots until they're almost translucent, about 3 minutes. Add the garlic and cook, stirring, for 1 minute, then add the Brussels sprouts. Increase the heat to medium-high and sauté the Brussels sprouts until tender, about 8 minutes. Stir in the lemon juice, then season to taste with salt and pepper. Transfer to a serving bowl.

Mango, Avocado, and Black Bean Salad **LYL**

This salad provides all the flavors of a Tex-Mex favorite without all the calories! The avocado provides satisfying fat, the fiber comes from the black beans, and the mango provides subtle sweetness.

SERVES 6

2 ripe but firm avocados, halved, peeled, pitted, and cubed
1 tablespoon freshly squeezed lime juice
2 ripe but firm mangoes, peeled, pitted, and cubed
1 (15-ounce) can no-added-salt black beans, drained and rinsed well

FOR THE LIME DRESSING
1 teaspoon grated lime zest
2 tablespoons freshly squeezed lime juice
2 tablespoons chopped fresh cilantro, plus more for garnish
½ teaspoon sea salt
¼ teaspoon freshly ground black pepper
¼ teaspoon sugar
3 tablespoons extra-virgin olive oil

Gently toss the avocado cubes with the lime juice in a medium-size bowl. Add the mangoes and gently toss to combine. Set aside.

Prepare the lime dressing: Whisk together the lime zest and juice, cilantro, salt, pepper, and sugar in a large bowl. Whisk in the olive oil until the mixture is thoroughly combined and creates a thick dressing. Add the avocado mixture and black beans and toss gently.

Spoon the salad onto individual plates, garnish with cilantro, and serve.

Mango Quinoa Salad🅢

With black beans and quinoa, this salad is substantial enough for a meal. With mango, coconut, and lime, it's equally refreshing!

SERVES 6

4 tablespoons white wine vinegar
3 tablespoons extra-virgin olive oil
1 tablespoon freshly squeezed lime juice
2 cups cooked quinoa, at room temperature
1 mango, seeded and diced
1 handful fresh cilantro, chopped
1 (15-ounce) can black beans, rinsed and drained
1 orange bell pepper, seeded and chopped
6 green onions or scallions, thinly sliced
3 tablespoons shredded unsweetened coconut

Whisk together the vinegar, olive oil, and lime juice in a small bowl.

Combine all the other ingredients, except the coconut, in a large bowl, then drizzle the dressing over the salad. Toss until the ingredients are thoroughly mixed, then chill for at least an hour. Top with the coconut right before serving.

Beet and Orange Salad 🄻🄨🄻

Roasting beets really brings out their sweetness; add oranges and quinoa for a salad that is light, healthy, and satisfying.

SERVES 4

Olive oil cooking spray
3 medium-size beets, peeled, trimmed, and diced
1⅓ cups uncooked quinoa, rinsed
1 tablespoon orange zest
2 oranges, peeled and sectioned (about 2 cups)
2 tablespoons chopped green onion or scallion, green part only
1 teaspoon extra-virgin olive oil

1 teaspoon white wine vinegar
Pinch each of sea salt and freshly ground black pepper

Heat the oven to 450°F. Spray a large roasting pan with olive oil cooking spray, and place the beets in the pan in a single layer. Cover the pan with foil and roast the beets in the oven for 15 minutes. Uncover the pan and roast the beets for another 10 minutes, or until tender when pierced with a fork. Remove from the oven and set aside to cool.

Meanwhile, bring 2 cups of water to a boil in a medium-pot over high heat. Pour in the quinoa, lower the heat to medium, cover the pot, and cook for 12 minutes. Remove from the heat, then fluff the quinoa with a fork.

Gently toss the diced beets with the orange zest and segments, onion, olive oil, vinegar, salt, and pepper in a large bowl.

To serve, place ¾ cup of the quinoa on individual plates, then top each with ¾ cup of the beet mixture.

Roasted Beet Salad🆂🅻

Complemented with tangy dressing on a bed of kale, the beets—which are high in many vitamins and minerals—are really allowed to shine in this simple salad.

SERVES 8

1½ pounds baby beets, leaves and stalks removed
1 head garlic
⅓ cup plus 2 tablespoons extra-virgin olive oil
½ teaspoon kosher salt
3 tablespoons red wine vinegar
1 teaspoon Dijon mustard
Sea salt and freshly ground black pepper
3 green onions or scallions, thinly sliced
6 cups torn kale, ribs removed
3 tablespoons finely chopped fresh cilantro

Preheat the oven to 325°F.

Rinse the beets thoroughly. Remove the excess papery skin from the garlic head without separating the cloves, then cut the head in half horizontally.

Toss the beets, garlic, 2 tablespoons of the olive oil, and the kosher salt in a small baking pan, then cover the pan with foil. Roast until tender, 1 to 1¼ hours. Remove from the oven and let the beets cool slightly.

Whisk together the vinegar and mustard in a medium-size bowl, then slowly add the remaining ⅓ cup of olive oil in a stream while continuing to whisk. Season the dressing to taste with sea salt and pepper. Squeeze the garlic cloves out of their skins into the bowl.

Peel and dice the beets, then add these to the bowl, along with the green onions, and toss to coat. Place the kale on a platter and top with the beet mixture. Garnish with the cilantro.

Warm Mushroom and Kale Salad LYL

Delicately flavored mushrooms pair with hearty kale for this filling—and healthful—salad.

SERVES 4

8 cups chopped kale, center ribs removed
2 tablespoons extra-virgin olive oil
1 large shallot, halved and sliced (about ½ cup)
3 cups sliced mixed mushrooms (such as shiitake, oyster, and cremini)
¼ teaspoon sea salt
¼ teaspoon freshly ground black pepper
2 tablespoons white balsamic vinegar
½ teaspoon honey

Place the kale in a large bowl and set aside.

Heat 1 tablespoon of the olive oil in a large skillet over medium heat, then add the shallot and cook, stirring, until translucent, 3 to 4 minutes. Add the mushrooms, salt, and pepper, and cook, stirring regularly, until the mushrooms are tender, 5 to 7 minutes.

Remove the skillet from the heat and stir in the remaining tablespoon of olive oil, the vinegar, and the honey, scraping up any browned bits.

Immediately pour the warm vinaigrette over the kale and toss to coat.

Kale Pesto and Barley Salad ⑤

A wonderful whole grain with nutty flavor and dense, chewy texture, barley is full of fiber and antioxidants. What better to pair it with than this dairy-free version of pesto—made from kale!

SERVES 4

1 cup whole-grain barley (about 8 ounces) (if you don't have barley, whole-grain couscous will work well)
2 tablespoons pine nuts
½ cup plus 2 tablespoons extra-virgin olive oil
1 tablespoon minced shallot
4 cups torn kale, center ribs removed
1 tablespoon freshly squeezed lemon juice
Kosher salt
2 tablespoons chopped preserved lemon (optional)

Cook the barley in salted boiling water in a medium-size saucepan over low heat until al dente, 30 to 45 minutes. Drain the barley well, transfer to a large bowl, and let cool slightly.

Meanwhile, toast the pine nuts in a small, dry skillet over low heat, stirring, until they're lightly golden, 3 to 5 minutes. Remove the pine nuts from the skillet and set aside.

In the same small skillet, heat 2 tablespoons of the olive oil, add the shallot, and cook over moderate heat, stirring, until golden, about

3 minutes. Scrape the shallot into the barley bowl and add the pine nuts.

Pulse two thirds of the kale along with the lemon juice in a food processor until the kale is chopped. With the machine running, slowly drizzle in the remaining ½ cup of olive oil and blend until the mixture is smooth. Season to taste with salt, then scrape the kale "pesto" into the barley mixture.

Add the preserved lemon, if using, and the remaining kale leaves. Season with additional salt, if desired, toss well, and serve.

Kale and Apple Salad **LYL**

Figs, apples, and pistachios add sweetness and texture to this elegant and easy salad—refreshing for lunch or as a side dish for dinner.

SERVES 6

3 tablespoons freshly squeezed lemon juice
2 tablespoons extra-virgin olive oil
¼ teaspoon kosher salt, plus more to taste
1 bunch kale, ribs removed, leaves very thinly sliced
¼ cup chopped dried figs
1 Honeycrisp apple
¼ cup chopped pistachios, toasted
Freshly ground black pepper

Whisk together the lemon juice, olive oil, and ¼ teaspoon of salt in a large bowl. Add the kale, toss to coat, and let stand for 10 minutes.

Meanwhile, cut the figs into thin slivers. Core the apple and slice into thin matchsticks.

Add the figs, apple, and pistachios to the kale. Season to taste with salt and pepper and toss well.

Zucchini and Farro Salad🟢

Protein and fiber-loaded farro pairs with vitamins A and C–rich zucchini for an easy warm salad with a touch of garlic.

SERVES 2

2 tablespoons olive oil
½ cup chopped Vidalia onion
1 tablespoon chopped fresh garlic
2 cups diced zucchini
½ teaspoon sea salt
¼ teaspoon coarsely ground black pepper
1 cup cooked farro

Heat the olive oil in a 12-inch sauté pan over medium heat, add the onion, and sauté until translucent, about 5 minutes.

Add the garlic and sauté for another minute, then add the zucchini, salt, and pepper and mix.

Add the farro and sauté until the mixture is thoroughly heated.

Dandelion Greens Salad with Sprouted Pumpkin Seeds 🟦

If you're new to dandelion greens, this salad is a wonderful introduction. Earthy, nutty, and with just a hint of bitterness, the greens are set off with the heartiness of pumpkin seeds and the sweetness of raisins.

SERVES 8

3 pounds dandelion greens, tough lower stems discarded, ribs and
    leaves cut diagonally into 2-inch pieces
½ cup extra-virgin olive oil
5 large garlic cloves, smashed
½ cup golden raisins
½ teaspoon fine sea salt
½ cup sprouted pumpkin seeds

Cook the greens in a 10- to-12-quart pot of boiling salted water, uncovered, until the ribs are tender, about 10 minutes. Drain in a colander, rinse under cold water to stop the cooking process, then drain well, gently pressing out any excess water.

Heat the olive oil in a 12-inch heavy skillet over medium heat until it shimmers, then cook the garlic, stirring, until it becomes pale gold. Add the raisins and cook, stirring, for about 45 seconds. Increase the heat to medium-high, then add the greens and salt and sauté until heated through, about 4 minutes. Place the salad in a serving bowl and sprinkle it with the sprouted pumpkin seeds.

Blackberry Freekeh Salad **LYL**

An ancient toasted grain, freekeh is nutty and crunchy. With antioxidant-heavy blackberries and Swiss chard, this salad is a delicious, hearty meal or side dish.

SERVES 4 TO 6

2 cups cooked freekeh, cooled
1 cup fresh blackberries
1½ cups chopped Swiss chard
½ cup slivered almonds
2 tablespoons olive oil
3 tablespoons freshly squeezed lemon juice
Sea salt and freshly ground black pepper

Combine the freekeh, blackberries, Swiss chard, and almonds in a large bowl and mix well.

Add the olive oil and lemon juice and toss to fully coat the ingredients.

Season to taste with salt and pepper.

Crispy Chickpea Salad⑤

Crispy chickpeas add a protein—and flavor—boost to this simple salad. If you don't have fig balsamic vinegar, regular will be just fine.

SERVES 1

1 tablespoon plus 1 teaspoon extra-virgin olive oil
½ cup mushrooms
½ cup Crispy Chickpeas (page 225)
2 cups torn or chopped kale leaves, ribs removed
2 teaspoons fig balsamic vinegar

Heat 1 teaspoon of the olive oil in a medium-size pan. Add the mushrooms and sauté until soft, about 7 minutes. Set aside.

Add the crispy chickpeas to the kale and stir in the mushrooms. Dress the salad with the remaining tablespoon of olive oil and the vinegar and toss until mixed well.

Chicken Salad⑤

A healthier twist on this lunchtime favorite! Swap traditional mayo for Vegenaise, an egg-free spread that's high in omega-3s. With garlic, mustard, and celery, you won't notice any difference in the taste.

SERVES 4

2 whole or 4 half chicken breasts, bone in, skin on
Olive oil
Kosher salt and freshly ground black pepper
½ cup Vegenaise
½ teaspoon Dijon mustard
1 teaspoon minced fresh garlic
1 cup diced celery (about 2 stalks)
1 cup green grapes, cut into quarters

Preheat the oven to 350°F.

Place the chicken breasts, skin side up, on a baking sheet, rub them with olive oil, and sprinkle generously with salt and pepper. Roast for 35 to 40 minutes, or until the chicken is cooked through. Set aside to cool.

When the chicken is cool, remove the meat from the bones and discard the skin and bones.

Dice the chicken into ¾-inch pieces and place in a bowl. Add the Vegenaise, mustard, garlic, celery, and grapes, plus 1½ to 2 teaspoons of salt and 1 teaspoon of pepper or to taste. Toss well, then refrigerate until ready to serve.

Albacore Tuna Salad ⓢ

Avocado is the secret ingredient here; mixed with yogurt or egg-free Vegenaise, spices, and topped on rice cakes, it makes for a light, refreshing meal or snack

SERVES 1

1 (5-ounce) can albacore tuna (packed in water)
½ medium-size avocado, peeled, pitted, and cut into chunks
¼ cup chopped red onion
1 tablespoon plain Greek yogurt or Vegenaise
½ teaspoon garlic salt
¼ teaspoon freshly ground black pepper
¼ cup chopped celery
½ cup seeded and chopped orange bell pepper
Juice of ½ lemon
1 teaspoon dried dill
½ teaspoon curry powder
½ teaspoon dried parsley
Brown rice cakes, for serving

Drain the tuna, place in a large bowl, and stir in the avocado chunks, red onion, yogurt, garlic salt, black pepper, chopped celery, and bell pepper. Mix well, then add the lemon juice, dill, curry powder, and parsley. Serve on top of brown rice cakes.

Wild Shrimp and Black Bean Salad ⑤

Mango and pineapple add a tropical note to this herb- and spice-rich dish. Serve it warm or cold—either way, it's delicious.

SERVES 4

¼ cup cider vinegar

3 tablespoons garlic-infused olive oil

1 tablespoon chili powder, or more to taste

1 teaspoon ground cumin

¼ teaspoon sea salt

1 pound peeled and deveined cooked wild shrimp, cut into ½-inch pieces

1 (15-ounce) can black beans, drained and rinsed

1 large orange bell pepper, seeded and chopped

¼ cup mango chunks

¼ cup pineapple chunks

¼ cup chopped green onion or scallion

¼ cup chopped fresh cilantro

Whisk together the vinegar, olive oil, chili powder, cumin, and salt in a large bowl. Add the shrimp, black beans, bell pepper, mango and pineapple chunks, green onion, and cilantro; toss to coat. Serve at room temperature or cold.

SALADS & SOUPS

Soups
Miso Soup with Spinach and Tofu
Black Bean Soup
Red Lentil Soup
Chickpea Stew
Curried Lentils
3-Bean Chili
Butternut Squash Soup
Easy Corn Soup

Note: All these soups freeze well, so make a double batch and store for a busy week. You can freeze individual servings for great grab-and-go healthy lunches.

Miso Soup with Spinach and Tofu (SL)

Just like the soup at your favorite Japanese restaurant, this recipe is easy, light, and filled with the probiotic goodness of miso and all the health benefits of sea vegetables.

SERVES 8

1 (12-ounce) block firm silken tofu
1 sheet nori (dried seaweed), cut into strips (about ¼ cup)
4 tablespoons white miso paste
4 green onions or scallions, thinly sliced
6 cups washed and torn or chopped spinach leaves
2 cups shredded carrot, for serving
2 cups shelled edamame, for serving

Wrap the block of tofu in two layers of paper towels and place it on a plate. Press down with your hands or a bowl to squeeze out any extra moisture, then cut the tofu into ¼- to ½-inch cubes.

Bring 4 cups of water to a simmer in a saucepan over medium heat, then add the nori and cook for 6 minutes.

In the meantime, whisk the miso paste in a bowl with some of the warm water from the pot until it's smooth, then add it to the pot. Add the tofu cubes, green onions, and spinach, and cook for another minute, or until all the ingredients are heated through.

Remove the soup from the heat and ladle it into eight bowls. Top each portion with ¼ cup of shredded carrot and ¼ cup of edamame. Serve immediately.

Black Bean Soup LYL

An easy and hearty soup with surprising ingredients: cinnamon—not only tasty, but long prized for its medicinal properties—and chia seeds, for an omega-3 boost.

SERVES 8

1 tablespoon olive oil
1 small onion, diced
1 pound dried black beans
12 cups vegetable stock
1 teaspoon garlic salt
1 teaspoon ground cumin
1 teaspoon ground cinnamon
2 tablespoons chia seeds, plus more if needed
1 cup low-fat plain Greek yogurt
⅓ cup chopped cilantro leaves and stems, as garnish

Heat the olive oil in a large pot over medium heat, then add the onion and sauté until translucent.

Add the black beans, vegetable stock, garlic salt, cumin, cinnamon, and chia seeds. Simmer, covered, for at least 2 hours, or until the beans are cooked.

If you want the soup thicker after cooking, add another tablespoon of chia seeds or blend half of the mixture with an immersion blender.

Serve with a dollop of Greek yogurt and chopped cilantro on top.

Red Lentil Soup LYL

Turmeric is an anti-inflammatory herb; mixed with ginger and other spices here, it creates a warming, hearty dish with flavors that deepen with each reheating.

SERVES 8

1 teaspoon olive oil
1 small yellow onion, chopped
1 cup finely chopped carrot
4 garlic cloves, chopped
1 teaspoon ground cumin
2 teaspoons ground turmeric
½ teaspoon ground ginger
1 teaspoon garam masala
Sea salt and freshly ground black pepper
5 cups vegetable stock
1½ cups dried red lentils
1 (29-ounce) can diced tomatoes, drained
¼ cup chopped fresh cilantro

Heat the olive oil in a large saucepan over medium heat for about 90 seconds, then add the onion and carrot and cook for 5 minutes, or until the onion is soft. Add the garlic and cook until it is lightly browned, then sprinkle in the cumin, turmeric, ginger, garam masala, and a pinch each of salt and pepper, stirring until the mixture is fragrant.

Mix in the vegetable stock, lentils, and tomatoes and bring to a simmer. Cover and cook for 20 minutes, until the lentils are tender.

Remove the pan from the heat and puree half of the soup, using a blender or an immersion blender. Pour the pureed soup back into the saucepan and stir in the cilantro.

Season to taste with salt and pepper, then serve.

Chickpea Stew⑤ℓ

Chickpeas are a versatile and tasty legume. Low in fat, high in fiber, they also help keep blood sugar levels stable—a miracle bean! Paired with spices and spinach, this satisfying stew will keep you feeling full without feeling stuffed.

SERVES 4

10 ounces baby spinach, washed
2 large garlic cloves, chopped
½ teaspoon sea salt
2 teaspoons chili powder
¼ teaspoon ground cumin
1 teaspoon curry powder or ground turmeric
¼ teaspoon freshly ground black pepper
2 (15-ounce) cans chickpeas, drained, liquid reserved
¼ cup extra-virgin olive oil
1 small sweet onion, finely chopped
1 large carrot, peeled and coarsely chopped
¼ cup golden raisins
½ cup chopped fresh parsley (optional)

Pour 1 cup of water into a large, deep skillet and bring it to a boil over high heat.

Add the spinach and cook, tossing frequently, until it has wilted, about 2 minutes.

Drain the spinach in a colander, pressing hard on the leaves to extract the liquid, then chop coarsely.

Mix the garlic with the salt in a small bowl, then add the chili powder, cumin, curry powder, and pepper, and mix until thoroughly combined. Stir in ¼ cup of the reserved chickpea liquid.

Wipe the skillet with a paper towel, then add 2 tablespoons of the olive oil to the skillet and heat for 1 minute. Add the onion and carrot to the skillet and cook over medium-high heat, stirring occasionally, until they are softened, about 3 minutes.

Add the spiced garlic mixture to the skillet and cook for 1 minute.

Add the chickpeas and the remaining chickpea liquid to the skillet, then stir in the raisins and bring the mixture to a boil over medium-high heat.

Add the spinach, lower the heat to medium, and simmer for 15 minutes.

Serve in a medium-size bowl and top with parsley, if desired.

Curried Lentils🆂🅛

If you've never cooked with lentils, you're in for a treat with this easy recipe. Lentils are packed with nutrition and are a good source of fiber, iron, potassium, and other minerals and vitamins. Add the liver-friendly ingredients curry powder and ginger and you've got a winning dish for lunch or dinner.

SERVES 4

3 tablespoons olive oil
2 garlic cloves, chopped
8 green onions or scallions, sliced, white and green parts separated
1 tablespoon curry powder
1 tablespoon ground ginger
1 large sweet potato (about 10 ounces), peeled and cut into 1-inch
   pieces
1 cup dried yellow lentils
4 cups low-sodium vegetable stock
¾ teaspoon sea salt
¼ teaspoon freshly ground black pepper
1 cup fresh cilantro (about a handful), chopped
4 tablespoons chopped peanuts

Heat the oil in a large saucepan over medium-high heat, then add the garlic and green onion whites. Cook, stirring frequently, until softened, 2 to 3 minutes.

Stir in the curry powder and ginger, add the sweet potato, lentils, stock, salt, and pepper, and bring the mixture to a boil.

Lower the heat and simmer, stirring occasionally, until the lentils and vegetables are tender, 15 to 20 minutes.

Sprinkle each serving with the cilantro, green onion greens, and 1 tablespoon of chopped peanuts.

3-Bean Chili⬤

This chili is so easy to make—you can whip it up on a weeknight (or on a weekend to freeze for later). With anti-inflammatory turmeric and omega-3-filled chia seeds, this delicious stew is as healthy as it is hearty.

SERVES 6 TO 8

¼ cup extra-virgin olive oil
1 yellow onion, chopped
1 to 2 tablespoons garlic cloves
1 tablespoon chia seeds
1 (14-ounce) can diced tomatoes
1 (15-ounce) can black beans, drained and rinsed
1 (15-ounce) can adzuki beans, drained and rinsed
1 (15-ounce) can pinto beans, drained and rinsed
1 (15-ounce can) vegetable stock
1 teaspoon sea salt
½ teaspoon freshly ground black pepper
½ teaspoon ground turmeric
1 (8-ounce) container plain full-fat Greek yogurt

Place the olive oil, onion, and garlic in a saucepan over medium heat and sauté for about 2 minutes, until the onion is translucent. Stir in 1 cup of water and the chia seeds, tomatoes, beans, vegetable stock, salt, pepper, and turmeric, and bring to a boil. Lower the heat and simmer for about 10 minutes further. If you desire a creamier texture, blend half of the mixture in a blender or with an immersion blender. Top each serving with 2 tablespoons of Greek yogurt.

Butternut Squash Soup℠

You can make this recipe with fresh, cooked squash, but to make it even easier, the ingredients calls for frozen. Nutmeg adds a delicate touch of spice. If you're vegetarian, you can swap in vegetable stock for the chicken stock.

SERVES 2 TO 4

1 tablespoon unsalted butter
2 carrots, diced
1 small yellow onion, chopped
3 cups chicken stock
1 (12-ounce) package frozen cooked squash
1 teaspoon freshly grated nutmeg
½ teaspoon sea salt
¼ teaspoon freshly ground black pepper
Fresh cilantro, as garnish

Place the butter, carrots, and onion in a saucepan over medium heat and sauté for about 2 minutes. Add the chicken stock, squash, nutmeg, salt, and pepper and bring to a boil, 2 to 3 minutes. Lower the heat and simmer for 5 more minutes, then turn off the heat and use an immersion blender to puree the entire soup mixture. Serve garnished with cilantro.

Easy Corn Soup 🄻🄻 ℠

Looking for a creamy soup you can enjoy, and not feel guilty about having? This one is it. It's filled with all the ingredients that help fight chronic disease in one delicious bowl. The soluble fiber in corn keeps you fuller and more satisfied, meaning you'll eat less at your next meal. The potassium helps in managing blood pressure by reducing the impact of sodium in the diet.

SERVES 4 TO 6

3 tablespoons olive oil
½ yellow onion
1 garlic clove, or 1 tablespoon crushed garlic
3 cups frozen corn kernels, defrosted

1½ cups vegetable stock
1 teaspoon ground cumin
1 teaspoon sea salt
½ teaspoon freshly ground black pepper
½ cup chopped parsley, for garnish (optional)

Heat the oil in a pot over medium heat, add and sauté the onion and garlic, then add the defrosted corn, vegetable stock, cumin, salt, and pepper and bring to a boil. Boil for 3 to 5 minutes. Remove and puree half of the mixture, using an immersion blender or standard blender. Return the pureed mixture to the pot, mix, and serve immediately. Garnish with the parsley.

SNACKS & SIDES

Hummus
Black Bean Hummus
White Bean Hummus
Edamame Hummus
Avocado Smear
Crispy Chickpeas
Brown Rice Balls
Sweet Potato Fries
Roasted Beet Chips
Roasted Root Vegetables
Baked Artichokes
Curried Cauliflower
Garlicky Tofu
Roasted Brussels Sprouts

Hummus **LYL** **SL**

Hummus is a terrific standby—it's great as a spread on whole-grain toast, crackers, or rice cakes; it's a dip that pairs with just about every veggie. This is a basic recipe; the secret is in the za'atar, a Middle Eastern spice blend, which adds a special savory kick. You can find tahini (ground sesame seed paste) at most grocery stores.

MAKES 4 CUPS HUMMUS

2 (15-ounce) cans chickpeas
1 tablespoon za'atar
7 large garlic cloves, unpeeled
½ cup extra-virgin olive oil
¼ teaspoon ground cumin, plus more for garnish
½ cup tahini, at room temperature
¼ cup plus 1 tablespoon freshly squeezed lemon juice
Sea salt
Paprika, for garnish
¼ cup chopped fresh parsley
Pita bread, for serving

Drain the chickpeas (reserving about ½ cup of the liquid) and rinse them under cold water. Place all but ½ cup of the chickpeas in a food processor (reserve the rest); add the za'atar, garlic, olive oil, cumin, tahini and lemon juice; and puree.

If you want a creamier texture, add a small amount of the reserved liquid from the chickpea can. Season the hummus to taste with salt and transfer it to a serving bowl.

Sprinkle the hummus with additional cumin and the paprika, and garnish it with the reserved whole chickpeas and the parsley. Serve with pita bread.

Black Bean Hummus SL

Out of chickpeas? You don't have to be out of hummus! This variation on the favorite spread has a Mexican-style flavor, with cumin and cilantro. Use it as a dip or as an accompaniment to Mexican meals.

SERVES 8

½ cup chopped fresh cilantro
2 tablespoons tahini
2 tablespoons freshly squeezed lemon juice
1 tablespoon extra-virgin olive oil
¾ teaspoon ground cumin
¼ teaspoon sea salt
1 (15-ounce) can no-added-salt black beans, drained and rinsed
1 garlic clove, peeled
2 teaspoons smoked paprika

Place 2 tablespoons of water, ¼ cup of the cilantro, and the tahini, lemon juice, olive oil, cumin, salt, black beans, and garlic in a food processor and process until smooth.

Spoon the hummus into a bowl and sprinkle with the remaining ¼ cup of cilantro. Top with the smoked paprika.

White Bean Hummus LYL

This has a similar flavor profile to chickpea hummus, with a delicious new taste of white beans. A perfect mash-up!

SERVES 6 TO 8

2 (15-ounce) cans navy beans, ½ cup of liquid reserved
¼ cup garlic-infused olive oil
½ cup tahini
2 tablespoons freshly squeezed lemon juice, plus more to taste (optional)
1 tablespoon soy sauce, plus more to taste (optional)
1 teaspoon ground cumin
Smoked paprika

Mix all the ingredients, except the smoked paprika, in a food processor, adding more lemon juice or soy sauce as needed. Sprinkle with smoked paprika.

Serve with 100% whole-grain pita chips, carrots, or celery sticks. This hummus also is a great condiment on sandwiches.

Edamame Hummus LYL SL

You may be most familiar with edamame as an appetizer at your favorite Japanese restaurant. This versatile bean also makes a great topping for salads—and here, another delicious riff on traditional hummus.

SERVES 4 TO 6

1 cup cooked edamame
¼ cup tahini
2 tablespoons freshly squeezed lemon juice
1 garlic clove, peeled
2 tablespoons olive oil
Sea salt

Combine the edamame, tahini, lemon juice, and garlic in a food processor and process until smooth.

Add the olive oil and continue to process the mixture until the oil is fully incorporated. Season to taste with salt, then serve.

Avocado Smear LYL

A hint of lemon, salt, and cumin take basic avocado to tasty heights. Use this as a spread on sandwiches, crackers, or rice cakes, or as a dip for veggies.

MAKES ABOUT 2 SERVINGS

1 ripe avocado, peeled and pitted
1 teaspoon freshly squeezed lemon juice
½ teaspoon garlic salt
2 teaspoons olive oil
1 teaspoon ground cumin

Mash the avocado in a medium-size bowl until smooth, then add the lemon juice, garlic salt, olive oil, and cumin.

Crispy Chickpeas LYL SL

These delicious bites are a great snack or topper for salads—especially the Crispy Chickpea Salad (page 211), where they're paired with kale, fig, and mushrooms.

SERVES 6 TO 8

2 (15-ounce) cans chickpeas
Olive oil
Sea salt
Paprika
Ground cumin

Preheat the oven to 425°F.

Rinse and drain the chickpeas, then pat them dry. Place in a single layer on a rimmed baking sheet and lightly drizzle with olive oil. Roast until the chickpeas are dark and crunchy, 30 to 40 minutes.

Remove from the oven, sprinkle to taste with salt, paprika, and cumin, then roast for a few more minutes.

Remove from the oven and allow the chickpeas to cool before serving. They can be stored in an airtight container in the fridge for about 3 days.

Brown Rice Balls ⑨

If you find yourself with leftover rice, whip up a batch of these flavorful gems. Similar to Japanese onigiri, *these are great to have on hand when you need a boost that's a bit of a heartier snack.*

MAKES 15 BALLS

2 cups cooked brown rice
1 cup finely chopped Swiss chard
1 medium-size green onion or scallion, chopped
2 tablespoons dried parsley
2 tablespoons tahini
½ teaspoon ground cumin
½ teaspoon garam masala
½ teaspoon paprika
Black sesame seeds, to coat

Mix all the ingredients, except the sesame seeds, in a bowl, then use your hands to form golf ball-size balls. Coat each ball with black sesame seeds. Set them aside at room temperature until ready to serve.

Sweet Potato Fries ⑨

Sweet potatoes are a great source of vitamins, including A and C; full of fiber and flavor, they make a great substitute for white potatoes. Missing French fries? These baked snacks are a great sandwich side.

MAKES 8 (1/2-CUP) SERVINGS

1½ tablespoons extra-virgin olive oil

1 tablespoon chopped fresh garlic

1 teaspoon sea salt

½ teaspoon freshly ground black pepper

2 pounds sweet potatoes, washed, peeled, and cut into small (¼-inch) sticks

1 teaspoon curry powder (optional)

Preheat the oven to 375°F.

Combine the olive oil with the garlic and seasonings in a large bowl. Add the potatoes and mix well, tossing until well coated.

Place in a single layer on a nonstick baking pan and bake for 35 minutes, or until tender.

Sprinkle with curry powder if you'd like a little more spice.

Roasted Beet Chips LYL

This recipe takes roasting root vegetables to the next level. Finely sliced beets are tossed in a delicate dressing and baked. Move over, potato chips!

SERVES 4

1 tablespoon extra-virgin olive oil

1 teaspoon minced fresh garlic

¼ teaspoon sea salt

⅛ teaspoon freshly ground black pepper

About 3 medium beets, peeled and cut into ⅛-inch slices (2 cups sliced)

Preheat the oven to 350°F.

Place all the ingredients, except the beets, in a medium-size bowl and mix thoroughly.

Place the beet slices in the oil mixture and toss thoroughly to coat.

Spread the beet slices in a single layer on a nonstick baking sheet. Roast in the oven for 25 minutes, or until the beets reach a desired degree of doneness. Consume within 2 days.

Roasted Root Vegetables 🆈

There's nothing quite like a hearty mix of roasted roots to accompany a salad or meal. They also make a great snack. While rutabaga and turnips may not be your go-tos, their sweetness comes out when lightly coated in olive oil, salt, and pepper, and roasted.

SERVES 6

½ cup extra-virgin olive oil
1 large red onion, thinly sliced
½ teaspoon sea salt
½ teaspoon freshly ground black pepper
1 cup peeled and diagonally sliced purple carrots
1 cup peeled and sliced rutabaga
1 cup peeled and sliced sweet potato (cut into thin rounds)
1 cup peeled and sliced turnip (cut into ½-inch wedges)

Preheat the oven to 375°F.

Heat 2 tablespoons of the olive oil in an ovenproof skillet over low heat, add the red onion slices, and season with ¼ teaspoon each of the salt and pepper. Sauté until the onion is golden brown, about 2 minutes, then remove from the heat and set aside.

In a 1-gallon resealable freezer bag, combine the vegetables and the remaining 6 tablespoons of oil, seal the bag, and shake it to thoroughly coat all the vegetables.

Add the vegetables to the sautéed onion and cover the pan with foil, poking a few holes in the foil with a fork to allow air to escape.

Roast in the oven for 35 to 45 minutes, or until the root vegetables are tender. Remove the foil and roast for an additional 15 minutes.

Roasted Brussels Sprouts LYL ⒮

If you've only had Brussels sprouts boiled, you are in for a treat. Roasting these mini cabbages removes any bitterness. With walnuts for extra omega-3s, this dish makes a great side for any meat-based meal.

SERVES ABOUT 4

Nonstick cooking spray
¼ cup extra-virgin olive oil
3 tablespoons fig balsamic vinegar (maple or cherry balsamic may be substituted)
1 teaspoon sea salt
½ teaspoon freshly ground black pepper
1 to 2 tablespoons crushed garlic
1 pound Brussels sprouts, washed, trimmed, and quartered
½ cup chopped walnuts

Preheat the oven to 425°F. Spray a large glass baking dish with cooking spray.

Whisk together the oil, balsamic vinegar, salt, pepper, and garlic in a medium-size bowl. Set aside.

Place the Brussels sprouts in a 1-gallon resealable plastic bag, add the oil mixture, and seal. Shake the bag to fully coat the sprouts and transfer the entire contents of the bag to the prepared baking dish.

Roast for 25 to 30 minutes. Remove from the oven and sprinkle the chopped walnuts on top. Bake for another 10 minutes, or until the sprouts are slightly browned.

Baked Artichokes 🆈🅻

You'll find it hard to believe a dish this tasty is so healthy. The cheese and panko add to the decadent nature of this dish—it's a great appetizer or accompaniment to an entrée, such as salmon and wild rice.

SERVES 4

1 cup whole wheat panko, toasted
1 tablespoon extra-virgin olive oil
1 tablespoon snipped fresh chives (½-inch lengths)
Juice of ½ lemon
1 garlic clove, minced
¼ cup grated Parmesan cheese
1 teaspoon kosher or sea salt
¼ teaspoon freshly ground black pepper
2 artichokes, trimmed

Preheat the oven to 400°F.

Combine the toasted panko, olive oil, chives, lemon juice, garlic, and Parmesan in a medium-size bowl, and season with ½ teaspoon of the salt and the pepper.

Cut off the top quarter of the artichokes lengthwise, spread the leaves of the artichoke, and pull out the center. Then, use a spoon to remove the bottom portion of the fuzzy choke, exposing only the leaves. Season the artichokes with ½ teaspoon of the salt.

Divide the panko mixture equally among the four artichoke halves, packing it into the cavities. Place the artichokes in a deep baking pan. Add about ½ inch of water and cover tightly with foil. Bake until the artichokes are tender and the panko is golden brown, about 1 hour.

Curried Cauliflower LYL

Cauliflower is the new kale! This versatile veg is a terrific base for these Indian-based flavors. Serve this dish alongside a light salad or lentil soup.

SERVES 4 TO 6

Nonstick cooking spray (optional)
2 teaspoons curry powder
1 teaspoon ground cumin
½ teaspoon chili powder
½ teaspoon sea salt
¼ teaspoon freshly ground black pepper
⅓ cup olive oil
1 medium-size head cauliflower, cut into florets
1 Vidalia onion, cut into eighths
½ cup chopped toasted walnuts

Preheat the oven to 425°F. Line a large baking sheet with foil or spray with nonstick cooking spray

Whisk together the curry powder, cumin, chili powder, salt, pepper, and olive oil in a medium-size bowl.

Spread the cauliflower florets and onion wedges in a single layer on the prepared baking sheet. Drizzle the spiced oil mixture over the vegetables and toss so they are thoroughly coated.

Roast the vegetables in the oven until they are tender and browned, about 40 minutes, turning halfway through cooking.

Serve hot or at room temperature in small bowls with 2 tablespoons of walnuts on top.

Garlicky Tofu 🄻🄮

Tofu is a great source of plant-based protein, providing about 9 grams for every 3 ounces. Better yet, studies show that soy may help to alleviate symptoms of fatty liver. Pair that with inflammation-fighting garlic and you've got a meal your liver will cheer about!

SERVES 4 TO 6

1 (14-ounce) package extra-firm tofu
3 tablespoons olive oil
3 tablespoons crushed garlic
Sea salt and freshly ground black pepper

Remove the tofu from the package and drain the water. Pat dry with paper towel and cut into 1-inch cubes. Place the tofu in a large bowl with 2 tablespoons of the olive oil, the garlic, and salt and pepper to taste. Mix thoroughly. In a separate pan, heat the remaining tablespoon of olive oil for 1 to 2 minutes, then add the tofu mixture. Sauté until the tofu is browned on all sides, 5 to 6 minutes. Serve immediately.

MAINS

Herb-Roasted Salmon with Brussels Sprouts

Salmon Arlene

Salmon Cakes

Cauliflower Steaks

Cauliflower-Crust Pizza

Chicken and Broccoli Pad Thai

Thai Peanut Spaghetti Squash

Portobello Mushroom Sandwiches

Chia Lentil Burgers

Spicy Turkey Burgers

Chia Turkey Meatballs

Spinach Turkey Meatballs

Chicken Stir-fry with Asparagus, Bell Peppers, and Cashews

Curried Tofu, Cashew, and Broccoli Stir-fry

Sesame Seed–Crusted Tofu

Lemony Soybean Spaghetti with Arugula

Green Bean and Quinoa Bowl

Creamy Peanut Quinoa Bowl with Sweet Potatoes

Swiss Chard Chicken Tacos

Fish Tacos

Tuna Patties

Easy Vegetable Pizza

Zucchini Pesto Pizza

Vegetable Frittata

Root Vegetable Gratin

Herb-Roasted Salmon with Brussels Sprouts ⓈⓁ

Garlic flavors this heart-healthy dish; the roasting brings out the flavor of both the fish and the nutritional-powerhouse Brussels sprouts.

SERVES 6

¼ cup garlic-infused olive oil
1 teaspoon sea salt
¾ teaspoon freshly ground black pepper
6 large garlic cloves
1 medium-size shallot, chopped
6 cups Brussels sprouts, trimmed and sliced
¾ cup white wine
2 pounds wild-caught salmon fillet, skinned, cut into 6 portions

Preheat the oven to 450°F.

Combine the garlic-infused olive oil, ½ teaspoon of the salt, and ¼ teaspoon of the pepper in a small bowl.

Halve the garlic cloves and toss them with the shallot, Brussels sprouts, and 3 tablespoons of the seasoned oil in a large roasting pan. Roast in the oven, stirring once, for 15 minutes.

Meanwhile, add the white wine to the remaining oil mixture. Remove the pan from the oven, stir the vegetables, and place the salmon fillets on top. Drizzle the fillets with the wine mixture, then lightly season each fillet with salt and pepper.

Bake the salmon until it is just cooked through, 5 to 10 minutes more.

Salmon Arlene ⓈⓁ

This healthy, omega-3-rich salmon dish was created by my mom (an incredible amateur chef), whose name is Arlene. She created it years ago and it has been a staple at Sunday night family dinners and birthdays ever since.

SERVES 4 TO 6

2 tablespoons olive or canola oil
1 medium-size onion, chopped
4 to 6 garlic cloves, chopped
¾ cup chopped fresh cilantro
¾ cup chopped fresh flat-leaf parsley
1½ to 2 pounds salmon fillet
Sea salt and freshly ground black pepper
1 cup white wine
2 cups chicken stock

Heat the oil in a large skillet over medium heat and sauté the onion and garlic until they're partially cooked, about 5 minutes. Add the cilantro and parsley.

Season the salmon with salt and pepper and place it, skin side up, on the onion mixture. Pour the white wine and chicken stock into the skillet until the salmon is almost covered.

Heat until the liquid is boiling, then cover the skillet with a lid, and lower the heat to low. Add more liquid as necessary to cover the salmon during cooking, 15 to 20 minutes.

Before serving, remove the skin and turn over the fillet onto a plate.

For a more flavorful and thicker sauce, continue to cook the sauce mixture down a bit, then cover the salmon with the sauce and serve.

Salmon Cakes ⑤ⓛ

These simple cakes make a satisfying meal when paired with brown rice and roasted vegetables or your favorite salad.

SERVES 4

Nonstick cooking spray
1 tablespoon extra-virgin olive oil
1 small red onion, finely chopped
2 tablespoons dried parsley
15 ounces canned wild salmon, drained, or 1½ cups cooked wild-
    caught salmon

1 large egg, lightly beaten
1½ teaspoons Dijon mustard
1¾ cups rolled oats
½ teaspoon freshly ground black pepper

Preheat the oven to 450°F. Coat a baking sheet with nonstick cooking spray and set aside.

Heat 1 ½ teaspoons of the olive oil in a large, nonstick skillet over medium-high heat. Add the red onion and cook, stirring, until softened, about 3 minutes. Stir in the parsley, then remove from the heat.

Place the salmon in a medium-size bowl and use a fork to flake it apart; remove any bones and skin. Add the egg and mustard and mix well, then add the onion mixture, oats, and pepper, mixing well. Shape the salmon mixture into eight patties, each about 2½ inches wide.

Heat the remaining 1½ teaspoons of olive oil in the pan over medium heat, add four salmon patties, and cook until their underside is golden, 2 to 3 minutes. Using a wide spatula, turn them over onto the prepared baking sheet. Repeat with the remaining patties.

Bake the salmon cakes until they're golden on top and heated through, 15 to 20 minutes. After cooking, pat off any excess oil with a paper towel.

Cauliflower Steaks LYL

Cauliflower is a vegetable that is truly hearty enough to be called "steak." Sliced thick and flavored with garlic and herbs, pair these substantial cuts with salad or protein, such as tofu or chicken breast.

MAKES 4 THICK "STEAKS"

1 head cauliflower
2 tablespoons garlic-infused olive oil
½ teaspoon sea salt
¼ teaspoon freshly ground black pepper

2 tablespoons dried parsley, or 3 tablespoons chopped fresh
1 tablespoon extra-virgin olive oil

Slice the cauliflower first down the center horizontally, then cut each half into two "steaks," keeping all four pieces, including the core, as intact as possible.

Place the garlic-infused olive oil in a ramekin, dip a brush in it, and brush both sides of the cauliflower steaks with the oil. Mix the salt, pepper, and parsley together in a small bowl and sprinkle over the steaks.

Heat a large, nonstick pan over medium-high heat, add the olive oil, and place the cauliflower steaks carefully in the pan. Sear the cauliflower steaks for 3 to 4 minutes per side, until they turn a deep golden color. Remove from the pan and serve.

Cauliflower-Crust Pizza ⑤

Yes, you can eat pizza while slimming your waist! The secret here is an oh-so-simple veg-based crust. Add your favorite toppings for a healthy twist on a classic favorite.

SERVES 6 TO 8

1 head cauliflower, stalk removed, or 1 (16-ounce) bag cauliflower crumbles)
¼ cup shredded mozzarella cheese
¼ cup grated Parmesan cheese
½ teaspoon garlic powder
1 tablespoon Italian seasoning
½ teaspoon sea salt
2 large eggs, lightly beaten
Possible toppings: chopped shallots, artichoke hearts, red onions, broccoli florets, tempeh chunks, olives, fresh kale or basil leaves

Preheat the oven to 400°F. Line a baking sheet with parchment paper and set aside.

Break the cauliflower into florets and pulse them in a food processor until fine (skip this step if you're using packaged cauliflower crumbles).

Place the cauliflower crumbles in a steamer basket and steam until tender. Drain well, transfer to a large bowl, and let cool.

Add the mozzarella, Parmesan, garlic powder, Italian seasoning, salt, and eggs to the cooled cauliflower, mixing thoroughly. Transfer the mixture to the center of the prepared baking sheet and spread it into a circle so that it resembles a pizza crust.

Bake for 20 minutes. Add whatever toppings you desire and bake for an additional 10 minutes.

Chicken and Broccoli Pad Thai⑤

This favorite Thai dish gets a healthy makeover, courtesy of edamame noodles.

SERVES 4

6 ounces edamame noodles
2 tablespoons peanut oil or sesame oil
3 garlic cloves, minced
½ cup egg whites, lightly beaten (from 3 large eggs)
8 ounces chicken breast, cut into bite-size pieces
2 cups broccoli florets
½ cup sliced green onion or scallion greens
¼ cup rice vinegar
2 tablespoons Asian fish sauce
1 tablespoon light brown sugar
½ teaspoon red pepper flakes
Chopped dry-roasted peanuts (optional)

Bring a large pot of water to a boil. Add the noodles and cook until they're just al dente, 5 to 6 minutes. Drain and set aside.

Heat 1 tablespoon of the oil in a wok or large, deep skillet over high heat, until the oil is very hot. Add the garlic and stir-fry until golden, about 10 seconds. Add the egg whites and cook, stirring, until scrambled, about 30 seconds.

Add the chicken pieces and remaining 1 tablespoon of oil; stir-fry until the chicken is cooked through and turns white, about 5 minutes. Add the noodles, broccoli florets, green onion greens, rice vinegar, fish sauce, brown sugar, and red pepper flakes and toss all the ingredients until heated through, 1 to 2 minutes.

If desired, sprinkle each serving with 1 tablespoon of peanuts before serving.

Thai Peanut Spaghetti Squash⑤

Luxurious coconut milk and peanut butter make a silky sauce—and a savory-sweet topping for squash, edamame, and broccoli.

SERVES 4

1 large spaghetti squash
1 tablespoon olive oil
Sea salt and freshly ground black pepper
½ cup no-added-sugar peanut butter
1 cup canned light coconut milk, plus more if needed
2 garlic cloves
1½ teaspoons ground ginger
1 tablespoon soy sauce
1½ teaspoons rice vinegar
1 large head broccoli, cut into bite-size florets and steamed
2 bunches Swiss chard, roughly chopped and steamed
1 cup cooked edamame
1 bunch green onions or scallions, chopped, for garnish
½ cup chopped peanuts, for garnish

Preheat the oven to 400°F. Line a baking sheet with foil and set aside.

Carefully cut the spaghetti squash in half lengthwise, using a large, sharp knife. Remove the seeds and stringy guts and discard or compost. Brush the cut insides of the squash with 1 tablespoon of the olive oil. Season with salt and pepper.

Place the spaghetti squash, cut side down, on the prepared baking sheet and roast until tender, 45 to 60 minutes. When it's done, the strands of the squash should fall off easily when scraped with a fork.

Remove from the oven and let the cooked spaghetti squash cool for about 5 minutes, then scrape all the flesh into a pile of strands in a large bowl. Taste and season with more salt and pepper, if needed.

Place the peanut butter, coconut milk, garlic, ginger, soy sauce, and rice vinegar in a blender, and blend on high speed until completely smooth; add a little more coconut milk if a thinner consistency is desired.

Mix the squash with the cooked broccoli, Swiss chard, and edamame. Divide equally among four bowls. Drizzle with the peanut sauce and sprinkle with the green onions and peanuts.

Portobello Mushroom Sandwiches 🆂🅻

Portobello mushrooms are a wonderful substitute for meat. Here, a quick grill and you have the foundation for a delicious sandwich you can load up with greens and avocado.

SERVES 4

1 small garlic clove, chopped
¼ cup Avocado Smear (page 225)
2 large or 3 medium-size portobello mushroom caps, gills removed
Olive oil cooking spray
½ teaspoon sea salt
½ teaspoon freshly ground black pepper
8 slices whole wheat bread, lightly grilled or toasted
2 cups washed and stemmed arugula or spinach (chop if large leaves)
1 large tomato, sliced

Preheat a grill to medium-high.

Use the back of a spoon to mash the garlic into a paste on a cutting board, then combine it with the avocado smear in a small bowl; set aside.

Coat both sides of the mushroom caps with olive oil cooking spray and season with the salt and pepper.

Grill the mushrooms, turning once, until they're tender and browned on both sides, 3 to 4 minutes. Remove from the heat.

When they're cool enough to handle, slice the mushrooms into three strips per cap.

Spread 1½ teaspoons of the avocado mixture on each piece of bread. Layer the mushrooms, arugula, and tomato slices atop the avocado on four slices of the bread and top with the remaining slices, avocado side down.

Chia Lentil Burgers LYL

Most veggie burgers fall down on the spot—literally! Here, the egg and rice bind the rest of the ingredients together for a patty that is substantial on the plate—and in your belly.

SERVES 8

1 tablespoon extra-virgin olive oil, plus more for baking sheet
1 cup chopped cremini mushrooms, chopped
1 medium-size onion, chopped
2 cups cooked steamed lentils
1 large egg
3 tablespoons soy sauce
1 cup cooked brown rice
1 cup chopped carrot
2 teaspoons ground cumin
1 cup chopped walnuts
½ cup chia seeds
1 tablespoon dried oregano
1 tablespoon dried parsley
2 garlic cloves, chopped

Preheat the oven to 400°F. Oil a baking sheet and set aside.

Heat the tablespoon of the olive oil in a medium-size saucepan over medium heat and sauté the mushrooms and onion until the onion is translucent.

Place 1 cup of the cooked lentils and the egg, soy sauce, and brown rice in a food processor and process until roughly pureed. Transfer the puree to a bowl and mix in the carrot, cumin, walnuts, chia seeds, oregano, parsley, garlic, and mushrooms mixture until well combined.

Mix in the remaining cup of lentils, form eight patties, place on the prepared baking sheet, and bake for about 25 minutes, or until the tops start to brown.

Spicy Turkey Burgers⬤

A combination of cinnamon, ginger, cayenne, and other spices amps up the flavor in these turkey burgers. Add tomato, spinach, and avocado and you've got a veggie-laden burger that can stand up with the best of 'em.

SERVES 4

2 teaspoons olive oil
½ cup seeded and chopped red bell pepper
2 garlic cloves, minced
1 teaspoon curry powder
½ teaspoon ground cumin
½ teaspoon ground cinnamon
½ teaspoon ground ginger
½ teaspoon sea salt
¼ teaspoon freshly ground black pepper
⅛ teaspoon cayenne pepper
1 teaspoon red pepper flakes
12 ounces ground turkey breast (all white meat)
1 cup cooked brown rice or quinoa
Nonstick cooking spray
4 whole wheat hamburger buns, split and toasted
½ cup Avocado Smear (page 225)

1 cup spinach leaves, washed
1 medium-size tomato, sliced

Heat the olive oil in a small, nonstick skillet over low heat for 1 to 2 minutes, then add the bell pepper, garlic, curry powder, cumin, cinnamon, ginger, salt, black pepper, cayenne, and red pepper flakes. Cook, stirring constantly, until the bell pepper is slightly softened, 1 to 2 minutes. Let cool.

Prepare a grill or preheat the broiler. Combine the turkey, brown rice, and pepper mixture in a medium-size bowl and mix thoroughly but lightly. Form four ¾-inch-thick patties. (Note: Because this burger is low in fat, you'll need to spray the grill or broiler pan with nonstick cooking spray before placing the patties on it.)

Grill or broil the patties until they have browned and are no longer pink inside, about 5 minutes per side. Serve each on a whole wheat bun with 2 tablespoons of avocado smear, topped with spinach leaves and sliced tomato.

Chia Turkey Meatballs ⓈⓁ

Whip up these protein- and nutrient-rich meatballs and serve over grain-free pasta with marinara sauce. Add a mixed green salad and you've got an easy, filling, classic meal.

SERVES 4

¼ cup black chia seeds
½ cup chicken stock
1 pound ground turkey breast (all white meat)
¾ cup whole wheat panko
½ cup chopped red onion
¼ cup grated Parmesan cheese
3 tablespoons basil-infused extra-virgin olive oil
½ teaspoon dried oregano
1½ teaspoons garlic salt
1 medium-size shallot, chopped
¼ teaspoon freshly ground black pepper

Preheat the oven to 350°F.

Combine the chia seeds and chicken stock in a large bowl; set aside and allow the chia seeds to swell for 15 minutes.

Meanwhile, combine the remaining ingredients in a large bowl and mix well, using your hands. Scoop or roll the meat mixture into meatballs about 1 inch in diameter.

Place the meatballs in a shallow baking pan and bake for 20 minutes, or until thoroughly cooked in the middle.

Remove from the oven and serve immediately.

Spinach Turkey Meatballs LYL

Adding spinach to these meatballs increases both the nutrition and the flavor. These are great served over whole wheat or grain-free spaghetti or rice with a side of veggies.

SERVES 4

Olive oil cooking spray
2 cups washed baby spinach
1 pound lean ground turkey
2 garlic cloves, minced
1 small shallot, finely chopped
1 large egg, lightly beaten
¾ cup whole-grain bread crumbs
½ cup grated Parmesan cheese
½ teaspoon sea salt
¼ teaspoon freshly ground black pepper

Preheat the oven to 450°F. Lightly spray a large baking dish with olive oil cooking spray and set aside.

Place a steamer basket over simmering water in a pot over medium heat and steam the baby spinach until it's wilted, 1 to 2 minutes. Let the spinach cool, squeeze out the water, and chop.

In a large bowl, combine the ground turkey, garlic, shallot, egg, bread crumbs, Parmesan, salt, pepper, and spinach; mix well. Use your hands to form the mixture into twelve equal-size meatballs.

Transfer the meatballs to the prepared baking dish and bake for 15 to 20 minutes, until the meatballs are golden brown and no longer pink inside.

Chicken Stir-fry with Asparagus, Bell Peppers, and Cashews **LYL**

The ancient grain freekeh makes a star appearance here as the base for this vegetable-friendly stir-fry. The slightly sweet sauce is offset with a little heat from the red pepper flakes.

SERVES 2 TO 4

1 tablespoon low-sodium soy sauce
1 tablespoon honey
2 boneless, skinless chicken breasts, cut into 1-inch pieces
1 tablespoon olive oil
1 bunch asparagus, cut into bite-size pieces
1 red bell pepper, seeded and chopped
1 orange bell pepper, seeded and chopped
½ cup whole cashews
4 garlic cloves, chopped
¼ teaspoon ground ginger
1 teaspoon red pepper flakes
2 teaspoons toasted sesame oil
2 cups cooked freekeh
½ cup chopped fresh cilantro, for garnish (optional)

Whisk together the soy sauce and honey in a medium bowl. Add the chicken pieces and stir to coat. Set the bowl in the refrigerator until you're ready to cook the chicken.

Meanwhile, heat the olive oil in a large skillet over medium-high heat. Add the asparagus and bell peppers, and sauté until cooked, about 5 minutes. Using a slotted spoon, remove the asparagus and peppers and set aside.

Remove the chicken from the marinade and add it to the skillet, reserving the marinade. Sauté until the chicken is nearly cooked through (with the insides still slightly pink), about 5 minutes. Then, add the cashews, garlic, ginger, red pepper flakes, and reserved marinade to the pan. Sauté for an additional 2 minutes, or until the chicken is fully cooked and the garlic is fragrant. Remove from the heat and stir in the sesame oil, asparagus, and peppers.

Serve immediately over ½ to 1 cup of freekeh per serving, garnished with cilantro, if desired.

Curried Tofu, Cashew, and Broccoli Stir-fry🅢

Tofu is a great chameleon, easily absorbing the flavors of sauces and marinades. Here, curry, garlic, and ginger combine with coconut milk for a healthy dish with a decadent taste.

SERVES 4

1 (14-ounce) package extra-firm water-packed tofu
3 tablespoons olive oil
1 tablespoon ground ginger
1 tablespoon curry powder
¼ teaspoon sea salt
2 tablespoons minced fresh garlic
1 (15-ounce) can light coconut milk
1 (4-ounce) jar red curry paste
6 cups broccoli florets, steamed
½ cup chopped cashews (optional)

Drain the tofu and press it between paper towels to remove any excess moisture before cutting it into 1-inch cubes.

Heat 2 tablespoons of the olive oil in a large pan over medium heat for 1 minute, then add the tofu cubes, ginger, curry powder, and salt. Cook until the tofu is golden, about 3 minutes on each side; set aside.

Heat the remaining olive oil in a medium-size pot, add the garlic and cook for 1 minute. Add the coconut milk and 3 to 4 tablespoons of red curry paste (depending on how hot you want it). Cook the sauce over low heat, mixing it well, for at least 5 minutes, or until the mixture appears red and creamy. Add the tofu and broccoli and mix well.

Remove from the heat and serve in small bowls, topping each with 2 tablespoons of chopped cashews, if desired.

Sesame Seed–Crusted Tofu ⓢⓛ

If you're new to cooking with tofu, this is a great starter recipe. The sesame seed–panko coating offers additional flavor and texture. Pair this with salad or veggies, such as roasted roots or broccoli, for an elegant meal.

SERVES 4

1 pound firm tofu, drained
¼ cup unsweetened almond milk
2 large egg whites, lightly beaten
½ teaspoon sea salt
¼ teaspoon freshly ground black pepper
3 tablespoons whole wheat panko
3 tablespoons black sesame seeds
½ teaspoon sesame oil or canola oil

Cut the tofu crosswise into twelve equal slices, then place the slices in a large, nonstick skillet over medium heat. Cook for 5 minutes on each side so that the tofu browns slightly and loses some of its liquid. Transfer to a plate and let it cool.

Whisk together the almond milk, egg whites, ¼ teaspoon of the salt, and the pepper in a medium bowl until well blended.

On a large plate, combine the panko, black sesame seeds, and remaining ¼ teaspoon of salt. Mix until well blended.

Dip a tofu slice into the milk mixture, then dredge it in the sesame seed mixture. Repeat the dipping and dredging with the remaining tofu slices.

Wipe out the skillet, then heat the sesame oil over medium heat. Arrange the tofu slices in the pan and cook, turning once, until lightly browned, about 3 minutes on each side. Transfer to a plate and keep warm until ready to serve.

Lemony Soybean Spaghetti with Arugula LYL

This recipe is so easy to whip up when you are craving something substantial but not heavy. Lemon and arugula complement each other for a light, bright flavor burst.

SERVES 4

12 ounces soybean spaghetti
1 tablespoon lemon-infused olive oil
½ cup grated Parmesan cheese, plus more for serving
1 teaspoon red pepper flakes
4 cups arugula
Sea salt and freshly ground black pepper

Bring a large pot of salted water to boil. Cook the spaghetti until al dente, 8 to 10 minutes. Drain, reserving 1 cup of the cooking liquid, and return the spaghetti to the pot. Add the lemon-infused olive oil, Parmesan, and ½ cup of the reserved cooking water to the pot and stir the ingredients gently to combine, adding cooking liquid as needed, until it's creamy.

Add the red pepper flakes and arugula and toss until the arugula just begins to wilt. Season to taste with salt and pepper, garnish with Parmesan, and serve.

Green Bean and Quinoa Bowl LYL

Nuts, greens, and protein, all in a flavorful bowl. Tuck into this healthy comfort food!

SERVES 2

2 tablespoons olive oil
½ cup chopped yellow onion
½ cup seeded and chopped yellow bell pepper
2 cups cooked green beans, cut into 1-inch pieces
½ teaspoon sea salt
½ teaspoon freshly ground black pepper
1 tablespoon minced fresh garlic
1 cup cooked quinoa
½ cup chopped raw almonds
½ cup watercress

Heat the olive oil in a medium-size pan over medium heat for 1 to 2 minutes, then add the onion and yellow pepper and cook for another 3 to 5 minutes. Add the green beans, salt, black pepper, and garlic and cook for another 2 minutes. Remove from the heat and place the entire mixture on the quinoa. Sprinkle the almonds and watercress on top.

Creamy Peanut Quinoa Bowl with Sweet Potatoes LYL

Sweet potatoes are loaded with vitamins and minerals. Not only are they healthy, they pair wonderfully with other vegetables and proteins. The creamy peanut dressing here brings out their sweetness.

SERVES 2

½ large sweet potato, peeled and cubed
1 tablespoon extra-virgin olive oil
Salt and freshly ground black pepper
½ head cauliflower, cut into florets
¼ cup quinoa, cooked
½ cup cubed tofu

DRESSING
2/3 cup light coconut milk
1 tablespoon pure maple syrup
2 tablespoons creamy no-added-sugar peanut butter

2 tablespoons lower-sodium soy sauce
⅛ teaspoon crushed red pepper

Preheat the oven to 400°F.

Place the cubed sweet potato on a baking sheet and toss with 1½ teaspoons of the olive oil; season with salt and pepper. Roast for 20 minutes. Remove from the oven, add the cauliflower florets to the baking sheet, toss them with the remaining 1½ teaspoons of olive oil, season with salt and pepper, and roast for an additional 20 minutes.

While the vegetables are roasting, whisk the dressing ingredients together in a bowl, then set aside.

Drain the tofu and press it between paper towels to remove any excess moisture, then cut it into 1-inch cubes.

When the vegetables are cooked, place the quinoa in individual bowls, top with the veggies and tofu, then drizzle 2 to 3 tablespoons of the dressing over each serving.

Swiss Chard Chicken Tacos **LYL**

The surprise healthy ingredient here? Chard leaves stand in as taco shells. Fill them with flavorful chicken and spinach for a new take on a Mexican classic.

SERVES 2 (3 TACOS PER SERVING)

1 tablespoon olive oil
1 medium-size onion, chopped
1 pound ground chicken breast
1 teaspoon garlic salt
1 teaspoon ground cumin
1 teaspoon garam masala
3 cups washed and chopped spinach
3 Swiss chard leaves, washed, red vein removed, each large strip cut in half horizontally

Heat the oil in a large skillet over medium-high heat and sauté the onion until translucent, about 2 minutes. Add the ground chicken, garlic salt, cumin, and garam masala and cook thoroughly, 6 to 8 minutes. Fold in the spinach and cook until it's wilted. Remove the skillet from the heat.

Use the Swiss chard leaves as "taco shells" for the chicken mixture.

Fish Tacos LYL

A simple, light, and refreshing taste of Baja! Tilapia is delicately seasoned and paired with fresh cabbage, beans, and salsa and nestled in corn tortillas.

SERVES 2

2 (4-ounce) frozen or fresh tilapia fillets
2 tablespoons low-sodium taco seasoning mix
4 (6-inch) whole corn tortillas
1 cup shredded cabbage
½ cup canned black beans, drained and rinsed
¼ cup low-fat Monterey jack cheese, shredded
Salsa (optional)
Corn (optional)
Hot sauce (optional)

Place the tilapia fillets in a nonstick pan, sprinkle them with the seasoning, and add ¼ cup of water. Cover the pan and cook over medium-high heat for 5 minutes, or until the fish is cooked thoroughly; remove from the heat.

Warm the tortillas in the microwave for 1 minute.

Flake the fish fillets. Onto each tortilla, spoon 2 ounces of the fish, ¼ cup of shredded cabbage, ¼ cup of black beans, and 1 tablespoon of shredded cheese.

Top with salsa and corn, if desired, and/or a splash of hot sauce.

Tuna Patties 🔲

These substantial burgers make a terrific lunch or dinner when placed in a whole-grain pita pocket and topped with veggies and sprouts. Or serve them with rice and a side of steamed broccoli or roasted veggies.

SERVES 6

4 (5-ounce) cans chunk light tuna in water, drained
1¼ cups 100% whole wheat panko or whole wheat bread crumbs
1 large egg, plus 2 large egg whites, lightly beaten
½ small sweet onion, finely chopped
2 tablespoons chopped fresh chives, green onion, or scallion
1 celery stalk, finely chopped
2 teaspoons Dijon mustard
2 teaspoons freshly squeezed lemon juice
2 garlic cloves, minced
½ teaspoon freshly ground black pepper
2 tablespoons olive oil

Preheat the oven to 200°F and place an ovenproof plate in the oven.

In a large bowl, combine all the ingredients, except the olive oil, and mix well. Use your hands to form the mixture into twelve ½-inch-thick patties; place the patties on a second plate.

Heat 1 tablespoon of the olive oil in a large skillet over medium-high heat. Working in batches, place the patties in the skillet in a single layer. Cook until golden brown on both sides, about 6 minutes total, flipping once or twice. Transfer the cooked patties to the plate in the oven.

Wipe out the skillet and repeat with the remaining oil and patties. Serve warm.

Easy Vegetable Pizza LYL

Everyone's favorite Friday night meal just got healthier with a whole-grain crust and loaded with veggies.

SERVES 4

1 (12-inch) 100% whole-grain pizza crust
Garlic-infused or plain extra-virgin olive oil
1 (14-ounce) jar water-packed artichoke hearts, drained and chopped
1 cup chopped broccoli
1 cup washed and torn or chopped spinach
1 garlic clove, chopped
1 cup shredded mozzarella cheese
1½ tablespoons dried oregano

Preheat the oven to 400°F. Brush the pizza crust with the olive oil. Spread the artichoke hearts, broccoli, spinach, garlic, and mozzarella evenly on top. Sprinkle with the oregano and bake for 20 minutes, or until the cheese is slightly browned on top. Cut into eight slices and serve.

Zucchini Pesto Pizza LYL

If you're a pesto lover, this easy pizza is for you. Mushrooms and zucchini complement the basil flavors and pack a nutritious punch.

SERVES 4

1 (12-inch) 100% whole wheat or 100% gluten-free corn pizza crust
½ cup pesto
1 to 2 zucchini, cut into strips
1 cup sautéed mushrooms
½ cup grated Parmesan cheese

Preheat the oven to 375°F. Brush the pizza crust with the pesto. Top with the zucchini strips, sautéed mushrooms, and Parmesan. Bake for 20 to 25 minutes, or until the crust is slightly browned. Cut into eight slices and serve.

Vegetable Frittata 🄻🄸🄻

This Spanish-Italian dish is so versatile: it makes a great brunch; or you can cook it up for dinner and serve it with salad—and take leftovers for lunch the following day. No matter when you eat it, it's nutritious, filling, and flavorful.

SERVES 4

2 large eggs, plus 4 large egg whites
¼ cup Parmesan cheese
1 teaspoon ground turmeric
½ cup seeded and chopped orange bell pepper
½ cup chopped red onion
1 teaspoon minced fresh garlic
½ teaspoon olive oil
2 cups washed and torn or chopped spinach
Sea salt and freshly ground black pepper

Whisk the eggs and egg whites in a medium-size bowl. Add the Parmesan, turmeric, bell pepper, red onion, and garlic; mix lightly. Heat the olive oil in nonstick pan over medium heat and add the egg mixture. Then, add the spinach leaves on top of the egg mixture. When the frittata is partially cooked (the perimeter of the eggs can be easily lifted with a spatula), place a plate on top of the egg mixture and flip the pan. Then, slide the opposite side of the mixture back into the pan to cook further until the egg mixture has solidified. Season to taste with salt and pepper and cut into four equal wedges.

Root Vegetable Gratin 🅂🄻

I developed this recipe with Chef Jim Perko. It's a great way to get less familiar root vegetables, such as parsnips and rutabaga, into your diet. This requires a little bit of work, but the rich flavors make it so worth it!

SERVES 6

2 teaspoons extra-virgin olive oil
2 cups firmly packed thinly sliced onion

½ teaspoon sea salt

½ teaspoon freshly ground black pepper

1 cup peeled and thinly sliced carrot (sliced on a long diagonal)

1 cup peeled and thinly sliced rutabaga

1 cup peeled and thinly sliced sweet potato (cut into rounds)

1 cup thinly sliced Idaho potatoes (cut into rounds)

1 cup peeled and thinly sliced parsnip (cut into lengthwise slices, core removed)

½ teaspoon smoked paprika

2½ cups vegetable stock

Preheat the oven to 375°F.

Heat the oil in a large skillet over a low heat. Add the onion and season with ¼ teaspoon each of the salt and pepper. Sauté until the onion is golden brown, then remove from the heat and set aside.

In an 8-inch square baking pan, create layers with each of the vegetables and the sautéed onion, seasoning each layer with salt, pepper, and smoked paprika. Repeat until all the vegetables, onion, and seasoning are used. Add the vegetable stock to the pan, cover (be sure to vent it), and place in the oven. Roast for 30 to 45 minutes. Remove the cover and cook for an additional 15 minutes. Note: The total cooking time will vary between 45 and 60 minutes, depending on the thickness of the cut vegetables and the desired degree of doneness.

SWEET TREATS
Chocolate Bark
Cinnamon Baked Almonds
Peanut Butter Balls
Vegan Truffles
Chocolate Espresso Tofu Mousse
Overnight Chia Seed Pudding
Pumpkin Bars
Avocado Brownie Bites

Chocolate Bark ⑤

Simple and full of antioxidants—what better way to enjoy a sweet treat?

MAKES 35 (1/2-OUNCE) SERVINGS

10 ounces dark or bittersweet chocolate (70% cacao), broken into
   pieces
½ cup toasted walnut pieces
½ cup toasted almond slices
¼ cup chopped apricots

Place the chocolate in a double boiler and heat over low heat, stirring, until almost fully melted. (Alternatively, melt the chocolate in a microwave by placing it in a small, microwave-safe bowl and microwaving it for 20 seconds at a time on MEDIUM, then stirring, until creamy.) Remove the chocolate from the heat and stir until smooth. Mix in the nuts and apricots.

Spread the mixture on a parchment paper–lined sheet pan and chill until set, about 30 minutes. Break into pieces and serve. Store in the fridge.

Cinnamon Baked Almonds ⑤

Almonds are truly a superfood. Here, they're a sweet treat with their light chocolate and cinnamon coating.

SERVES 8 TO 10

Nonstick cooking spray
1 large egg white
3 cups almonds
4 teaspoons ground cinnamon
3 tablespoons unsweetened cocoa powder

Preheat the oven to 400°F. Line a baking or cookie sheet with foil and spray with nonstick cooking spray.

Lightly beat the egg white in a bowl. Add the almonds and toss until they're well coated; sprinkle the cinnamon and cocoa onto the almonds and stir to coat evenly.

Spread the nuts in a single layer on the prepared baking sheet. Bake for 10 minutes, stirring halfway through the baking time.

Remove the baking sheet from the oven and carefully separate the nuts by hand so they won't be clumped together. Store them in an airtight container.

Peanut Butter Balls **LYL**

A healthy snack that's also the perfect mix of nutty and sweet.

MAKES 15 TO 18 BALLS

½ cup dried apricots
2 cups natural, unsalted, crunchy peanut butter
2 tablespoons ground flaxseeds
1 tablespoon amber honey

Chop the apricots and place in a medium-size bowl. Mix in the rest of the ingredients. Transfer the mixture to the freezer for 1 hour to set.

After removing from the freezer, use your hands or a melon baller to shape the mixture into small balls. Store them in the refrigerator.

Vegan Truffles ᴸʸᴸ

Chocolate. Coconut. Nuts. Yes, giving your liver a little love does involve these three decadent ingredients!

MAKES 16

9 ounces (1¼ cups) vegan dark chocolate (72% cacao or higher), finely chopped or grated

7 tablespoons light coconut milk, well mixed

½ cup unsweetened coconut flakes

3 tablespoons chopped walnuts

Place the chocolate in a medium-size, heatproof bowl.

Pour the coconut milk into a small, microwave-safe bowl and microwave on MEDIUM-HIGH until it's very warm but not boiling, about 25 seconds. (Alternatively, heat in a small saucepan over medium heat until it starts to simmer.)

Immediately add the coconut milk to the chocolate and loosely cover the bowl with a pot lid or towel to trap in the heat; let it sit for 5 minutes, then lift the cover and use a mixing spoon to gently stir until the chocolate is completely melted, creamy, and smooth. Place the mixture in the refrigerator and chill, uncovered, for 2 to 3 hours, or until it's almost completely solid.

Once the mixture is firm, mix the coconut flakes and chopped walnuts together on a small plate for rolling. Use a tablespoon or melon baller to shape the mixture into small balls, then use your hands to gently but quickly roll them in the coconut mixture.

Shake off the excess, then place the truffles on a parchment paper–lined serving dish. Serve immediately or refrigerate until ready to serve.

Chocolate Espresso Tofu Mousse ⓢⓛ

If you think taking chocolate out of your diet is essential to healthy living and weight loss, think again. It's the type of chocolate that matters most. This recipe is one of my favorites from Chef Jim Perko. It uses chocolate with a high cocoa content and that's key when it comes to getting the flavonoids that chocolate delivers. One study even showed that cocoa could help fight against inflammation and reduce liver triglycerides. This recipe can be made with decaffeinated coffee to reduce the overall caffeine.

MAKES 12 (1/4-CUP) SERVINGS

12 ounces extra-firm tofu
2 ripe bananas
6 tablespoons unsweetened cocoa powder
5 teaspoons real maple syrup or agave nectar
2 teaspoons pure vanilla extract
2 ounces bittersweet chocolate (70% cacao)
2 tablespoons instant espresso powder

Place the tofu in a food processor and blend until creamy. Add the bananas and process until smooth.

Add the cocoa powder, agave nectar, and vanilla and process until thoroughly mixed.

Prepare a saucepan of simmering water while shaving the chocolate into thin pieces.

Place the chocolate shavings and espresso powder in a medium-size glass or metal bowl. Place the bowl on top of the saucepan of simmering water.

Use a rubber spatula to mix the chocolate as it begins to melt. Promptly remove the bowl from the pot once the chocolate has melted. Be careful—the bowl will be hot!

Add the melted chocolate to the tofu mixture and process until smooth.

Transfer to individual dishes or a large bowl.

Overnight Chia Seed Pudding ⑤ᴸ

You can use this versatile recipe to start your day (it's a nourishing breakfast—consider adding fruit), take an afternoon snack break, or finish your evening meal. No matter when you eat it, this creamy tapioca-like pudding is a real treat.

SERVES 4

1 cup vanilla-flavored unsweetened almond milk
1 cup plain low-fat or fat-free Greek yogurt
1 tablespoon pure maple syrup
1 teaspoon pure vanilla extract
⅛ teaspoon sea salt
¼ cup chia seeds
¼ cup sliced almonds
¼ cup chopped walnuts

Gently whisk the almond milk, yogurt, maple syrup, vanilla and salt in a medium-size bowl until just blended. Whisk in the chia seeds, then let the mixture stand for 30 minutes; stir gently if the seeds begin to settle. Cover and refrigerate overnight.

The next day, mix in the almonds and walnuts, then spoon the pudding into four bowls or glasses and serve.

Pumpkin Bars ᴸʸᴸ

These dense, moist bars are sweet enough to satisfy a craving, but not so sweet to send you into a sugar rush. Bonus: There are no refined grains in this recipe, only nutrient-rich ingredients that make a treat that's not only delicious, but also a snack that will give you energy and keep you going.

MAKES 7 LARGE BARS

1 (8-ounce) package dates
¾ cup walnuts
¾ cup almonds
¾ cup peanuts
3 tablespoons hemp seeds

1 tablespoon pure maple syrup
2 tablespoons pure pumpkin puree
½ cup unsweetened shredded coconut
1 teaspoon pure vanilla extract
1½ teaspoons ground cinnamon
1½ teaspoons ground allspice

Place all the ingredients in a food processor and continuously pulse until the mixture is thoroughly combined but some chunks of nuts remain.

Line a 9-inch square pan with parchment paper, leaving an inch or two of overhang of paper on two opposite sides for easy lifting. Spread the mixture in the prepared pan, using a spatula to firmly press it down against the bottom of the pan. Allow it to set for 30 minutes in the refrigerator, then use the paper overhang to lift the entire slab out of the pan. Cut into bars.

Avocado Brownie Bites `LYL`

You may be surprised at the secret ingredient here: avocado, which deepens the chocolate flavor and adds creaminess. These bites are so rich and decadent, you won't need more than one to be satisfied!

MAKES 16 SMALL BROWNIE BITES

Nonstick cooking spray
1 ripe avocado, peeled and pitted
4 tablespoons butter, melted
1 large egg
½ cup light brown sugar
½ cup pure maple syrup
2 teaspoons pure vanilla extract
¾ cup unsweetened cocoa powder
¼ teaspoon sea salt
1¼ cups gluten-free flour
½ cup dark chocolate chips, melted

Preheat the oven to 350°F. Spray an 8-inch square baking pan with nonstick cooking spray.

Mash the avocado in a large bowl until smooth, then add the melted butter, egg, brown sugar, maple syrup, vanilla, and 2 teaspoons of water. Mix well to combine. Add the cocoa powder and stir until fully incorporated and free of any large lumps.

Combine the flour and salt in a separate bowl, then stir in the avocado mixture and melted chocolate. Spread the batter evenly in the prepared pan and bake for 35 to 40 minutes, until the brownies are cooked through. Allow the brownies to cool in the pan before cutting them into 16 brownie bites.

appendix b
metric conversions chart

The recipes in this book have not been tested with metric measurements, so some variations might occur.

Remember that the weight of dry ingredients varies according to the volume or density factor: 1 cup of flour weighs far less than 1 cup of sugar, and 1 tablespoon doesn't necessarily hold 3 teaspoons.

General Formulas for Metric Conversion

Ounces to grams	>	ounces × 28.35 = grams
Grams to ounces	>	grams × 0.035 = ounces
Pounds to grams	>	pounds × 453.5 = grams
Pounds to kilograms	>	pounds × 0.45 = kilograms
Cups to liters	>	cups × 0.24 = liters
Fahrenheit to Celsius	>	(°F − 32) × 5 ÷ 9 = °C
Celsius to Fahrenheit	>	(°C × 9) ÷ 5 + 32 = °F

Weight (Mass) Measurements

1 ounce = 30 grams
2 ounces = 55 grams
3 ounces = 85 grams
4 ounces = ¼ pound = 125 grams
8 ounces = ½ pound = 240 grams
12 ounces = ¾ pound = 375 grams
16 ounces = 1 pound = 454 grams

Volume (Liquid) Measurements

1 teaspoon = 1/6 fluid ounce = 5 milliliters
1 tablespoon = ½ fluid ounce = 15 milliliters
2 tablespoons = 1 fluid ounce = 30 milliliters
¼ cup = 2 fluid ounces = 60 milliliters
1/3 cup = 2 2/3 fluid ounces = 79 milliliters
½ cup = 4 fluid ounces = 118 milliliters
1 cup or ½ pint = 8 fluid ounces = 250 milliliters
2 cups or 1 pint = 16 fluid ounces = 500 milliliters
4 cups or 1 quart = 32 fluid ounces = 1,000 milliliters
1 gallon = 4 liters

Oven Temperature Equivalents, Fahrenheit (F) and Celsius (C)

100°F = 38°C
200°F = 95°C
250°F = 120°C
300°F = 150°C
350°F = 180°C
400°F = 205°C
450°F = 230°C

Volume (Dry) Measurements

¼ teaspoon = 1 milliliter
½ teaspoon = 2 milliliters
¾ teaspoon = 4 milliliters
1 teaspoon = 5 milliliters
1 tablespoon = 15 milliliters
¼ cup = 59 milliliters
1/3 cup = 79 milliliters
½ cup = 118 milliliters
2/3 cup = 158 milliliters
¾ cup = 177 milliliters
1 cup = 225 milliliters
4 cups or 1 quart = 1 liter
½ gallon = 2 liters
1 gallon = 4 liters

Linear Measurements

½ inch = 1½ cm
1 inch = 2½ cm
6 inches = 15 cm
8 inches = 20 cm
10 inches = 25 cm
12 inches = 30 cm
20 inches = 50 cm

appendix c
stress-trigger tracking sheet

Stressor	Your Response to the Stress	Your Physical Symptoms	Your Coping Actions
(This could be a person, an event, an ongoing situation like caring for an ill family member, or an isolated incident, such as someone cutting you off in traffic.)	(What was your immediate reaction? Did you yell or get upset? Did you try to bury your feelings?)	(What physical symptoms occurred due to the stress? Did your stomach ache? Did you get a headache or muscle and joint pain? Were your symptoms brief or long lasting?)	(After the stressful event, what did you do to manage your feelings? Did you try to numb them by drinking alcohol or eating sweets? Did you try to improve your mind-set by taking a walk or meditating? What tools helped you get through the situation?)

appendix d
healthy liver weekly journal

Week of _____
Weight _____

Action Step	Challenges	Notes
Consumed at least 5 fruits and vegetables every day		
Made all of my grains whole grains		
Avoided added sugars		
Consumed healthy fats		
Consumed lean sources of protein with meals		
Kept alcohol consumption within recommended ranges		
Avoided sugary beverages and consumed water, tea, or coffee		
Physical activity for at least 30 minutes daily		
Engaged in stress management techniques		
Slept at least 7 hours each night		

acknowledgments

Writing a book is a challenging endeavor. It's actually quite similar to changing stubborn habits to improve your health in that if you do it alone, you will most likely not succeed, but if you surround yourself with people that care for you and have your back—then you can thrive. This book could not have been possible without the people that shaped me, the people that stood by me, and the people that loved me throughout the course of my life and my career. I'd like to start with my husband, Andy. For your unwavering support, your guidance, your love, your wonderful humor, your ability to make difficult tasks and situations seem easy and your love of our children. You are my everything. Thank you for being a be*liver* in me. I love you more than words will ever express. For my mother, Arlene, and my father, Irving. As a nurse and a physician, you taught me at an early age the importance and the power of helping others heal their health. As my mom and dad, you gave me confidence, unconditional love, a clear moral compass and every opportunity to be who I wanted to be. I am the woman I am today because of the both of you, and this book is a testament to all you said I could achieve if I worked hard enough. I love you both! For my friend and agent, Bonnie Solow, who believed in me from the start, and who guided me through the unpredictable road of publishing better than anyone ever could have done. You are amazing; if everyone had a Bonnie to walk next to them in life, we'd all have a more clear vision of the road ahead. For writer Stacey Colino, your talent is unbelievable! For always keeping me on track, and for teaching me how to take complicated medical information and translate it into something that everyone can not only appreciate, but enjoy as well. For my editor, Renée Sedliar, you have the incredible ability of taking a good chapter and turning it into something remarkable and even magical. Thank you for the countless hours spent making this book what it is. For Dr. Ibrahim Hanouneh, for your friendship, for your medical expertise, and for your always positive and warm personality. You truly exemplify what it means to be a compassionate physician. Your patients are lucky to know you. So am I. For my brothers, Jeff and Brian; being the baby sister of two older brothers made me one tough cookie. Thank you for that; it helped shape who I became and gave me strength and courage when I needed it the most. I love you both. For my mentors, whom I have been privileged to work with, especially Dr. Michael Roizen, Dr. Mladen Golubic, Dr. Paul Terpaluk, Dr. Richard Lang, Dr. Mehmet Oz, Dr. Michael O'Donnell, Dr. Stacey Snelling, and the late Dr. Tanya Edwards. You have shown me what it means to work hard and to truly care about those you serve in your profession, but even more remarkably, you taught me how to treat those who stand beside you with grace, respect and above all, appreciation. Thank you for your encouragement and your guidance in helping make me a better caregiver. It has been an honor to work alongside you. For the most amazing dietitians I have ever known who I get to call friends and colleagues, especially Laura Jeffers, Brigid Titgemeier, Ashley Koff, Christina Palmisano, Julia Zumpano, Amy Jones, Jasmine El Nabli, and Beth Bluestone. For my friends, who supported me 100 percent and had at times been forced to endure hours upon hours of "book talk" but who still loved me despite it! Especially Carlynn and Hank Schlissberg, Toya and Joe Gorley, Mia Ferrara, Sonya Taylor, Danielle Pirain, Rita Petti, Mimy Tong, Beth Grubb, Jennifer DeGrant, Charles DeSantis (and his wagon), and Jamie Starkey. For the Cleveland Clinic Corporate Communications team and my Wellness Institute team, especially Scott Katsikas, Regina Chandler, Jim Perko, Judi Bar, and Jane Ehrman, and for Cleveland Clinic CEO Dr. Toby Cosgrove, who had the vision to make wellness a priority at the Cleveland Clinic. Finally, for all the countless patients and individuals not mentioned here who have touched my life in one way or another. People come into our lives for very different reasons but in the end, they all shape our decisions throughout our journey on this earth. Deciding to write this book was perhaps one of the biggest in my life. Thank you for playing a part in that.

—Kristin Kirkpatrick

The most beautiful thing in this world is to see your patients smiling, and knowing that your work is the reason behind that smile. I hope this book brings a smile on your face, and helps you tackle the new silent epidemic—fatty liver disease.

It brings me a great pleasure for the opportunity to work on the "Skinny Liver" project. For this I'm deeply indebted and sincerely thankful to my friend and author, Kristin Kirkpatrick, for invaluable guidance and elating encouragement throughout the course of present work.

I would like to express my special thanks to our editor, Renée Sedliar, literary agent, Bonnie Solow, and writer, Stacey Colino. The completion of this project could not have been possible without their assistance and that of so many people whose names may not all be encountered. Their contribution is sincerely appreciated and greatly acknowledged.

To my parents, who have been a source of encouragement and inspiration throughout my life.

To my siblings, Dima and Mo, whose value to me only grows with age.

To my mentor, Dr. Nizar Zein, who guided me through the various stages of my career. There is no one quite like a special teacher and no teacher quite as special as you.

My appreciation also extends to the Cleveland Clinic, and to my patients who taught me that the reward for work well done is the opportunity to do more.

I'm grateful beyond measure to you all.

—Ibrahim Hanouneh

Both Ibrahim and I would also like to thank the team at Perseus/Da Capo for their dedication to this book—some key folks here who have been "behind the scenes," but have been instrumental supporters of the book include Susan Weinberg, John Radziewicz, Kevin Hanover, Lissa Warren, Miriam Riad, Isabelle Bleecker, and Jennifer Thompson. And of course, Christine Marra, for whom we give thanks daily!

selected references

Abd El-Kader, S. M., O. H. Al-Jiffri, and F. M. Al-Shreef. 2014. "Liver Enzymes and Psychological Well-being Response to Aerobic Exercise Training in Patients with Chronic Hepatitis C." *African Health Sciences* 14 (2) (June): 414-19.

Abdelmalek, M. F., A. Suzuki, C. Guy, A. Unalp-Arida, R. Colvin, R. J. Johnson, and A. M. Diehl. 2010. "Increased Fructose Consumption Is Associated with Fibrosis Severity in Patients with Nonalcoholic Fatty Liver Disease." *Hepatology* 51 (6) (June): 1961-71.

Ajmera, V. H., E. P. Gunderson, L. B. VanWagner, C. E. Lewis, J. J. Carr, and N. A. Terrault. 2016. "Gestational Diabetes Mellitus Is Strongly Associated with Non-Alcoholic Fatty Liver Disease." *American Journal of Gastroenterology* 111 (5) (May): 658-64.

Albano, E., E. Mottaran, G. Occhino, E. Reale, and M. Vidali. 2005. "Review Article: Role of Oxidative Stress in the Progression of Non-alcoholic Steatosis." *Alimentary Pharmacology and Therapeutics* 22 (s2) (November): 71-73.

Ali, A. A., M. T. Velasquez, C. T. Hansen, A. I. Mohamed, and S. J. Bhathena. 2004. "Effects of Soybean Isoflavones, Probiotics, and Their Interactions on Lipid Metabolism and Endocrine System in an Animal Model of Obesity and Diabetes." *Journal of Nutritional Biochemistry* 15 (10) (October): 583-90.

Aller, R., D. A. De Luis, O. Izaola, R. Conde, M. Gonzalez Sagrado, D. Primo, B. De La Fuente, and J. Gonzalez. 2011. "Effect of a Probiotic on Liver Aminotransferases in Nonalcoholic Fatty Liver Disease Patients: A Double Blind Randomized Clinical Trial." *European Review for Medical and Pharmacological Sciences* 15 (9) (September): 1090-95.

American Liver Foundation. "Alcohol-Related Liver Disease." http://www.liverfoundation.org/abouttheliver/info/alcohol/.

American Liver Foundation. "The Progression of Liver Disease." http://www.liverfoundation.org/abouttheliver/info/progression/.

Askari, F., B. Rashidkhani, and A. Hekmatdoost. 2014. "Cinnamon May Have Therapeutic Benefits on Lipid Profile, Liver Enzymes, Insulin Resistance, and High-Sensitivity C-Reactive Protein in Nonalcoholic Fatty Liver Disease Patients." *Nutrition Research* 34 (2) (February): 143-48.

Assunção, M., M. J. Santos-Marques, R. Monteiro, I. Azevedo, J. P. Andrade, F. Carvalho, and M. J. Martins. 2009. "Red Wine Protects Against Ethanol-Induced Oxidative Stress in Rat Liver." *Journal of Agricultural and Food Chemistry* 57 (14): 6066-73.

Ayala, A., M. F. Muñoz, and S. Argüelles. 2014. "Lipid Peroxidation: Production, Metabolism, and Signaling Mechanisms of Malondialdehyde and 4-Hydroxy-2-Nonenal." *Oxidative Medicine and Cellular Longevity.* http://dx.doi.org/10.1155/2014/360438.

Azzalini, L., E. Ferrer, L. N. Ramalho, M. Moreno, M. Domínguez, J. Colmenero, V. I. Peinado, J. A. Barberà, V. Arroyo, P. Ginès, J. Caballería, and R. Bataller. 2010. "Cigarette Smoking Exacerbates Nonalcoholic Fatty Liver Disease in Obese Rats." *Hepatology* 51 (5) (May): 1567-76.

Bahirwani, R., and K. R. Reddy. 2009. "Outcomes After Liver Transplantation: Chronic Kidney Disease." *Liver Transplantation,* Supplement S2 (November): S70-S74.

Behm, D. G., A. J. Blazevich, A. D. Kay, and M. McHugh. 2016. "Acute Effects of Muscle Stretching on Physical Performance, Range of Motion, and Injury Incidence in Healthy Active Individuals: A Systematic Review." *Applied Physiology, Nutrition, and Metabolism* 41: 1-11.

Behrens, G., C. E. Matthews, S. C. Moore, N. D. Freedman, K. A. McGlynn, J. E. Everhart, A. R. Hollenbeck, and M. F. Leitzmann. 2013. "The Association Between Frequency of Vigorous Physical Activity and Hepatobiliary Cancers in the NIH-AARP Diet and Health Study." *European Journal of Epidemiology* 28 (1) (January): 55-66.

Bellentani, S., G. Saccoccio, F. Masutti, L. S. Crocè, G. Brandi, F. Sasso, G. Cristanini, and C. Tiribelli. 2000. "Prevalence of and Risk Factors for Hepatic Steatosis in Northern Italy." *Annals of Internal Medicine* 132 (2) (January 18): 112-17.

Birerdinc, A., M. Stepanova, L. Pawloski, and Z. M. Younossi. 2012. "Caffeine Is Protective in Patients with Non-alcoholic Fatty Liver Disease." *Alimentary Pharmacology & Therapeutics* 35 (1) (January): 76-82.

Blais, P., N. Husain, J. R. Kramer, M. Kowalkowski, H. El-Serag, and F. Kanwal. 2015. "Nonalcoholic Fatty Liver Disease Is Underrecognized in the Primary Care Setting." *American Journal of Gastroenterology.* 110 (1) (January): 10-14.

Browning, J. D., J. A. Baker, T. Rogers, J. Davis, S. Satapati, and S. C. Burgess. 2011. "Short-Term Weight Loss and Hepatic Triglyceride Reduction: Evidence of a Metabolic Advantage with Dietary Carbohydrate Restriction." *American Journal of Clinical Nutrition* 93 (5): (May) 1048-52.

Buettner, D. 2008. *The Blue Zones: Lessons for Living Longer from the People Who've Lived the Longest.* Washington, DC: National Geographic.

Bugianesi, E., E. Gentilcore, R. Manini, S. Natale, E. Vanni, N. Villanova, E. David, M. Rizzetto, and G. Marchesini. 2005. "A Randomized Controlled Trial of Metformin Versus Vitamin E or Prescriptive Diet in Nonalcoholic Fatty Liver Disease." *American Journal of Gastroenterology.* 100 (5) (May): 1082-90.

Cani, P. D., A. M. Neyrinck, F. Fava, C. Knauf, R. G. Burcelin, K. M. Tuohy, G. R. Gibson, and N. M. Delzenne. 2007. "Selective Increases of Bifidobacteria in Gut Microflora Improve High-Fat-Diet-Induced Diabetes in Mice Through a Mechanism Associated with Endotoxaemia." *Diabetologia* 50 (11) (November): 2374-83.

Capanni, M., F. Calella, M. R. Biagini, S. Genise, L. Raimondi, G. Bedogni, G. Svegliati-Baroni, F. Sofi, S. Milani, R. Abbate, C. Surrenti, and A. Casini. 2006. "Prolonged N-3 Polyunsaturated Fatty Acid Supplementation Ameliorates Hepatic Steatosis in Patients with Non-alcoholic Fatty Liver Disease: A Pilot Study." *Alimentary Pharmacology & Therapeutics* 23 (8) (April 15): 1143-51.

Carey, E., A. Wieckowska, and W. D. Carey. 2013. "Nonalcoholic Fatty Liver Disease" Cleveland Clinic Center for Continuing Education (March). http://www.clevelandclinicmeded.com/medicalpubs/diseasemanagement/hepatology/nonalcoholic-fatty-liver-disease/Default.htm.

Cassidy, S., C. Thoma, K. Hallsworth, J. Parikh, K. G. Hollingsworth, R. Taylor, D. G. Jakovljevic, and M. I. Trenell. 2016. "High Intensity Intermittent Exercise Improves Cardiac Structure and Function and Reduces Liver Fat in Patients with Type 2 Diabetes: A Randomized Controlled Trial." *Diabetologia* 59 (1) (January): 56-66.

Cave, M., S. Appana, M. Patel, K. C. Falkner, C. J. McClain, and G. Brock. 2010. "Polychlorinated Biphenyls, Lead, and Mercury Are Associated with Liver Disease in American Adults: NHANES 2003-2004." *Environmental Health Perspectives* 118 (12) (December): 1735-42.

Chang, A.-M., D. Aeschbach, J. F. Duffy, and C. A. Czeisler. 2015. "Evening Use of Light-Emitting eReaders Negatively Affects Sleep, Circadian Timing, and Next-Morning Alertness." *PNAS* 112 (4) (January 27); 1232-37.

Chida, Y., N. Sudo, and C. Kubo. 2006. "Does Stress Exacerbate Liver Diseases?" *Journal of Gastroenterology and Hepatology* 21 (1): 202-8.

Chiu, A. 2008. "Jeremy Piven's Doc: Star Stricken by Toxins from Sushi." *People*, December 18, 2008. http://www.people.com/people/article/0,,20247781,00.html.

Cho, J. Y., T. H. Chung, K. M. Lim, H. J. Park, and J. M. Jang. 2014. "The Impact of Weight Changes on Nonalcoholic Fatty Liver Disease in Adult Men with Normal Weight." *Korean Journal of Family Medicine* 35 (5) (September): 243-50.

Chou, T. C., W. M. Liang, C. B. Wang, T. N. Wu, and L. W. Hang. 2015. "Obstructive Sleep Apnea Is Associated with Liver Disease: A Population-Based Cohort Study." *Sleep Medicine* 16 (8) (August): 955-60.

Chrousos, G. P. 1995. "The Hypothalamic-Pituitary-Adrenal Axis and Immune-Mediated Inflammation." *New England Journal of Medicine* 332 (May 18): 1351-63.

Collier, J. 2007. "Non-alcoholic Fatty Liver Disease." *Medicine* 35 (2) (February): 86–88.

Cooper, C. C. 2009. "Nonalcoholic Fatty Liver Disease—Strategies for Prevention and Treatment of an Emerging Condition." *Today's Dietitian* 11 (12) (December): 28.

Corbin, K. D., and S. H. Zeisel. 2012. "Choline Metabolism Provides Novel Insights into Nonalcoholic Fatty Liver Disease and Its Progression." *Current Opinion in Gastroenterology* 28 (2) (March): 159–65.

Corey, K. E., J. Misdraji, L. Gelrud, L. Y. King, H. Zheng, A. Malhotra, and R. T. Chung. 2015. "Obstructive Sleep Apnea Is Associated with Nonalcoholic Steatohepatitis and Advanced Liver Histology." *Digestive Diseases and Sciences* 60 (8) (August): 2523–28.

Cresswell, J. D., L. E. Pacilio, E. K. Lindsay, and K. W. Brown. 2014. "Brief Mindfulness Meditation Training Alters Psychological and Neuroendocrine Responses to Social Evaluative Stress." *Psychoneuroimmunology* 44 (June): 1–12.

De Filippis, F., N. Pellegrini, L. Vannini, I. B. Jeffery, A. La Storia, L. Laghi, D. I. Serrazanetti, R. Di Cagno, I. Ferrocino, C. Lazzi, S. Turroni, L. Cocolin, P. Brigidi, E. Neviani, M. Gobbetti, P. W. O'Toole, and D. Ercolini. 2015. "High-Level Adherence to a Mediterranean Diet Beneficially Impacts the Gut Microbiota and Associated Metabolome." *Gut* (September 28). http://gut.bmj.com/content/early/2015/09/03/gutjnl-2015-309957.abstract.

Dennis, E. A., A. L. Dengo, D. L. Comber, K. D. Flack, J. Savla, K. P. Davy, and B. M. Davy. 2010. "Water Consumption Increases Weight Loss During a Hypocaloric Diet Intervention in Middle-Aged and Older Adults." *Obesity* 18 (2) (February): 300–307.

Dongiovanni, P., R. Rametta, M. Meroni, and L. Valenti. 2016. "The Role of Insulin Resistance in Nonalcoholic Steatohepatitis and Liver Disease Development—A Potential Therapeutic Target?" *Expert Review of Gastroenterology & Hepatology* 10 (2): 229–42.

Dunn, W., R. Xu, and J. B. Schwimmer. 2008. "Modest Wine Drinking and Decreased Prevalence of Suspected Nonalcoholic Fatty Liver Disease." *Hepatology* 47 (6) (June): 1947–54.

Eguchi, Y., Y. Kitajima, H. Hyogo, H. Takahashi, M. Kojima, M. Ono, N. Araki, K. Tanaka, M. Yamaguchi, T. Eguchi, K. Anzai, and Japan Study Group for NAFLD. 2015. "Pilot Study of Liraglutide Effects in Non-alcoholic Steatohepatitis and Non-alcoholic Fatty Liver Disease with Glucose Intolerance in Japanese Patients." *Hepatology Research* 45 (3) (March): 269–78.

Emery, C. F., K. L. Olson, V. S. Lee, D. L. Habash, J. L. Nasar, and A. Bodine. 2015. "Home Environment and Psychosocial Predictors of Obesity Status Among Community-Residing Men and Women." *International Journal of Obesity* 39:1401–7.

Environmental Working Group. 2016. *2016 Shopper's Guide to Pesticides in Produce.* https://www.ewg.org/foodnews/summary.php.

Fang, R., and X. Li. 2015. "A Regular Yoga Intervention for Staff Nurse Sleep Quality and Work Stress: A Randomized Controlled Trial." *Journal of Clinical Nursing* 24 (23-24) (December): 3374-79.

Farhangi, M. A., B. Alipour, E. Jafarvand, and M. Khoshbaten. 2014. "Oral Coenzyme Q10 Supplementation in Patients with Nonalcoholic Fatty Liver Disease: Effects on Serum Vaspin, Chemerin, Pentraxin 3, Insulin Resistance and Oxidative Stress." *Archives of Medical Research* 45 (7) (October) 589-95.

Farsi, F., M. Mohammadshahi, P. Alavinejad, A. Rezazadeh, M. Zarei, and K. A. Engali. 2016. "Functions of Coenzyme Q10 Supplementation on Liver Enzymes, Markers of Systemic Inflammation, and Adipokines in Patients Affected by Nonalcoholic Fatty Liver Disease: A Double-Blind, Placebo-Controlled, Randomized Clinical Trial." *Journal of the American College of Nutrition* 35 (4) (May-June): 346-53.

Feldstein, A. E., P. Charatcharoenwitthaya, S. Treeprasertsuk, J. T. Benson, F. B. Enders, and P. Angulo. 2009. "The Natural History of Non-alcoholic Fatty Liver Disease in Children: A Follow-up Study for up to 20 Years." *Gut* 58 (11) (November): 1538-44.

Fisher, C. D., A. J. Lickteig, L. M. Augustine, R. P. J. Oude Elferink, D. G. Besselsen, R. P. Erickson, and N. J. Cherrington. 2009. "Experimental Non-alcoholic Fatty Liver Disease Results in Decreased Hepatic Uptake Transporter Expression and Function in Rats." *European Journal of Pharmacology* 613 (1-3) (June 24): 119-27.

Food and Drug Administration. "BPA: Reducing Your Exposure." http://www.fda.gov/forconsumers/consumerupdates/ucm198024.htm.

Framson, C., A. R. Kristal, J. Schenk, A. J. Littman, S. Zeliadt, and D. Benitez. 2009. "Development and Validation of the Mindful Eating Questionnaire." *Journal of the American Dietetic Association* 109 (8) (August): 1439-44.

Francois, M. E., J. C. Baldi, P. J. Manning, S. J. E. Lucas, J. A. Hawley, M. J. A. Williams, and J. D. Cotter. 2014. "'Exercise Snacks' Before Meals: A Novel Strategy to Improve Glycaemic Control in Individuals with Insulin Resistance." *Diabetologia* 57 (7) (July): 1437-45.

Geng, T., A. Sutter, M. D. Harland, B. A. Law, J. S. Ross, D. Lewin, A. Palanisamy, S. B. Russo, K. D. Chavin, and L. A. Cowart. 2015. "SphK1 Mediates Hepatic Inflammation in a Mouse Model of NASH Induced by High Saturated Fat Feeding and Initiates Proinflammatory Signaling in Hepatocytes." *Journal of Lipid Research* 56 (12) (December): 2359-71.

Ghaemi, A., F. A. Taleban, A. Hekmatdoost, A. Rafiei, V. Hosseini, Z. Amiri, R. Homayounfar, and H. Fakheri. 2013. "How Much Weight Loss Is Effective on Nonalcoholic Fatty Liver Disease?" *Hepatitis Monthly* 13 (12) (December): e15227.

Gooley, J. J., K. Chamberlain, K. A. Smith, S. B. Khalsa, S. M. Rajaratnam, E. Van Reen, J. M. Zeitzer, C. A. Czeisler, and S. W. Lockley. 2011. "Exposure to Room Light Before Bedtime Suppresses Melatonin Onset and Shortens Melatonin Duration in Humans." *Journal of Clinical Endocrinology and Metabolism* 96 (3) (March): E463-E72.

Gothe, N. P., and E. McAuley. 2015. "Yoga Is as Good as Stretching-Strengthening Exercises in Improving Functional Fitness Outcomes: Results from a Randomized Controlled Trial." *Journals of Gerontology Series A: Biological Sciences and Medical Sciences.* http://biomedgerontology.oxfordjournals.org/content/early/2015/08/21/gerona.glv127.long

Grant, B. J., D. A. Dawson, F. S. Stinson, S. P. Chou, M. C. Dufour, and R. P. Pickering. 2004. "The 12-Month Prevalence and Trends in DSM-IV Alcohol Abuse and Dependence: United States, 1991-1992 and 2001-2002." *Drug and Alcohol Dependence* 74:223-34.

Greenfield, T. K., L. T. Midanik, and J. D. Rogers. 2000 "A 10-Year National Trend Study of Alcohol Consumption, 1984-1995: Is the Period of Declining Drinking Over?" *American Journal of Public Health* 90 (1) (January): 47-52.

Guicciardi, M. E., and G. J. Gores. 2005. "Apoptosis: A Mechanism of Acute and Chronic Liver Injury." *Gut* 54:1024-33.

Hallsworth, K., G. Fattakhova, K. G. Hollingsworth, C. Thoma, S. Moore, R. Taylor, C. P. Day, and M. I. Trenell. 2011. "Resistance Exercise Reduces Liver Fat and Its Mediators in Non-alcoholic Fatty Liver Disease Independent of Weight Loss." *Gut* 60 (9) (September): 1278-83.

Harrison, S. A., and C. P. Day. 2007. "Benefits of Lifestyle Modification in NAFLD." *Gut* 56 (12) (December): 1760-69.

Harrison, S. A., W. Fecht, E. M. Brunt, and B. A. Neuschwander-Tetri. 2009. "Orlistat for Overweight Subjects with Nonalcoholic Steatohepatitis: A Randomized, Prospective Trial." *Hepatology* 49 (1) (January): 80-86.

Heden, T., C. Lox, P. Rose, S. Reid, and E. P. Kirk. 2011. "One-Set Resistance Training Elevates Energy Expenditure for 72 h Similar to Three Sets." *European Journal of Applied Physiology* 111 (3) (March): 477-84.

Helander, E. E., A. L. Vuorinen, B. Wansink, and I. K. Korhonen. 2014. "Are Breaks in Daily Self-Weighing Associated with Weight Gain?" *PLoS One* 9 (11) (November 14): e113164.

Henao-Mejia, J., E. Elinav, C. Jin, L. Hao, W. Z. Mehal, T. Strowig, C. A. Thaiss, A. L. Kau, S. C. Eisenbarth, M. J. Jurczak, J. P. Camporez, G. I. Shulman, J. I. Gordon, H. M. Hoffman, and R. A. Flavell. 2012. "Inflammasome-Mediated Dysbiosis Regulates Progression of NAFLD and Obesity." *Nature* 482 (7384) (February 1): 179-85.

Hultcrantz, R., H. Glaumann, G. Lindberg, and L. H. Nilsson. 1985. "Liver Investigation in 149 Asymptomatic Patients with Moderately Elevated Activities of Serum Aminotransferases." *Scandinavian Journal of Gastroenterology* 21 (1) (January): 109-13.

Hyogo, H., T. Ikegami, K. Tokushige, E. Hashimoto, K. Inui, Y. Matsuzaki, H. Tokumo, F. Hino, and S. Tazuma. 2011. "Efficacy of Pitavastatin for the Treatment of Non-alcoholic Steatohepatitis with Dyslipidemia: An Open-Label, Pilot Study." *Hepatology Research* 41 (11) (November): 1057-65.

Institute for Functional Medicine. 2010. *The Textbook of Functional Medicine.*

Integrated Medicine Institute. "Heavy Metals: Mercury and Lead Damage to theLiver."http://www.imi.com.hk/heavy-metals-mercury-and-lead-damage -liver-the-rising-prevalence-of-fatty-liver-disease-is-partly-due-to-heavy -metal-exposure.html.

Ishitobi, T., H. Hyogo, H. Tokumo, K. Arihiro, and K. Chayama. 2014. "Efficacy of Probucol for the Treatment of Non-alcoholic Steatohepatitis with Dyslipidemia: An open-label pilot study." *Hepatology Research.* 44 (4) (April): 429-35.

Jackson, S. E., A. Steptoe, and J. Wardle. 2015. "The Influence of Partner's Behavior on Health Behavior Change: The English Longitudinal Study of Ageing." *JAMA Internal Medicine* 175 (3): 385-92.

Jamal, H. Z. 2015. "Non-Alcoholic Fatty Liver Disease: America's Greatest Health Risk of 2015?" *Scientific American*, February 9. http://blogs. scientificamerican.com/guest-blog/non-alcoholic-fatty-liver-disease -america-s-greatest-health-risk-of-2015/.

Jin, X., R. H. Zheng, and Y. M. Li. 2008. "Green Tea Consumption and Liver Disease: A Systematic Review." *Liver International* 28 (7) (August): 990-96.

Johnson, N. A., T. Sachinwalla, D. W. Walton, K. Smith, A. Armstrong, M. W. Thompson, and J. George. 2009. "Aerobic Exercise Training Reduces Hepatic and Visceral Lipids in Obese Individuals Without Weight Loss." *Hepatology* 50 (4) (October): 1105-12.

Jollow, D. J., S. S. Thorgeirsson, W. Z. Potter, M. Hashimoto, and J. R. Mitchell.1974. "Acetaminophen-Induced Hepatic Necrosis. VI. Metabolic Disposition of Toxic and Nontoxic Doses of Acetaminophen." *Pharmacology* 12 (4-5): 251-71.

Kavanagh, K., A. T. Wylie, K. L. Tucker, T. J. Hamp, R. Z. Gharaibeh, A. A. Fodor, and J. M. Cullen. 2013. "Dietary Fructose Induces Endotoxemia and Hepatic Injury in Calorically Controlled Primates." *American Journal of Clinical Nutrition* 98 (2) (August): 349-57.

Keating, S. E., D. A. Hackett, H. M. Parker, H. T. O'Connor, J. A. Gerofi, A. Sainsbury, M. K. Baker, V. H. Chuter, I. D. Caterson, J. George, and N. A. Johnson. 2015. "Effect of Aerobic Exercise Training Dose on Liver Fat and Visceral Adiposity." *Journal of Hepatology* 63 (1) (July): 174-82.

Kechagias, S., A. Ernersson, O. Dahlqvist, P. Lundberg, T. Lindström, and F. H. Nystrom. 2008. "Fast-Food-Based Hyper-alimentation Can Induce Rapid and Profound Elevation of Serum Alanine Aminotransferase in Healthy Subjects." *Gut* 57 (5) (May): 649-54.

Keyworth, C., J. Knopp, K. Roughley, C. Dickens, S. Bold, and P. Coventry. 2014. "A Mixed-Methods Pilot Study of the Acceptability and Effectiveness of a

Brief Meditation and Mindfulness Intervention for People with Diabetes and Coronary Heart Disease." *Behavioral Medicine* 40 (2) (April): 53-64.

Klein, E. A., I. M. Thompson Jr., C. M. Tangen, J. J. Crowley, M. S. Lucia, P. J. Goodman, L. M. Minasian, L. G. Ford, H. L. Parnes, J. M. Gaziano, D. D. Karp, M. M. Lieber, P. J. Walther, L. Klotz, J. K. Parsons, J. L. Chin, A. K. Darke, S. M. Lippman, G. E. Goodman, F. L. Meyskens Jr., and L. H. Baker. 2011. "Vitamin E and the Risk of Prostate Cancer: The Selenium and Vitamin E Cancer Prevention Trial (SELECT)." *JAMA* 306 (14) (October 12): 1549-56.

Kohli, R., M. Kirby, S. A. Zanthakos, S. Softic, A. E. Feldstein, V. Saxena, P. H. Tang, L. Miles, M. V. Miles, W. F. Balistreri, S. C. Woods, and R. J. Seeley. 2010. "High-Fructose Medium-Chain-Trans-Fat Diet Induces Liver Fibrosis and Elevates Plasma Coenzyme Q9 in a Novel Murine Model of Obesity and NASH." *Hepatology* 52 (3) (September): 934-44.

Kondo, Y., T. Kato, O. Kimura, T. Iwata, M. Ninomiya, E. Kakazu, M. Miura, T. Akahane, Y. Miyazaki, T. Kobayashi, M. Ishii, N. Kisara, K. Sasaki, H. Nakayama, T. Igarashi, No Obara, Y. Ueno, T. Morosawa, and T. Shimosegawa. 2013. "1(OH) Vitamin D3 Supplementation Improves the Sensitivity of the Immune-Response During Peg-IFN/RBV therapy in Chronic Hepatitis C Patients—Case Controlled Trial." *PLoS One* 8 (5) (May 23): e63672.

Kong, A., S. A. A. Beresford, C. M. Alfano, K. E. Foster-Schubert, M. L. Neuhouser, D. C. Johnson, C. Duggan, C.-Y. Wang, L. Xiao, R. W. Jeffery C. E. Bain, and A. McTiernan. 2012. "Self-Monitoring and Eating-Related Behaviors Associated with 12-Month Weight Loss in Postmenopausal Overweight-to-Obese Women." *Journal of the Academy of Nutrition and Dietetics* 112 (9) (September): 1428-35.

Koopman, K. E., M. W. A. Caan, A. J. Nederveen, A. Pels, M. T. Ackermans, E. Fliers, S. E. laFelur, and M. J. Serlie. 2014. "Hypercaloric Diets with Increased Meal Frequency, but Not Meal Size, Increase Intrahepatic Triglycerides: A Randomized Controlled Trial." *Hepatology* 60 (2) (August): 545-53.

Kwak, M. S., D. Kim, G. E. Chung, W. Kim, Y. J. Kim, and J. H. Yoon. 2015. "Role of Physical Activity in Nonalcoholic Fatty Liver Disease in Terms of Visceral Obesity and Insulin Resistance." *Liver International* 35 (3) (March): 944-52.

Lassailly, G., R. Caiazzo, D. Buob, M. Pigeyre, H. Verkindt, J. Labreuche, V. Raverdy, E. Leteurtre, S. Dharancy, A. Louvet, M. Romon, A. Duhamel, F. Pattou, and P. Mathurin. 2015. "Bariatric Surgery Reduces Features of Nonalcoholic Steatohepatitis in Morbidly Obese Patients." *Gastroenterology* 149 (2) (August): 379-88.

Lata, R. P., and B. V. Verma. 2015. "A Study of the Effect of Yogic Package on Blood Profile of Alcoholics." *International Journal of Yoga and Allied Sciences* 4 (1) (January-June): 28-30.

Leach, N. V., E. Dronca, S. C. Vesa, D. P. Sampelean, E. C. Craciun, M. Lupsor, D. Crisan, R. Tarau, R. Rusu, I. Para, and M. Grigorescu. 2014. "Serum Homocysteine Levels, Oxidative Stress and Cardiovascular Risk in Non-alcoholic Steatohepatitis." *European Journal of Internal Medicine* 25 (8) (October): 762-67.

"Lean Patients with Fatty Liver Disease Have Higher Mortality Rate." 2014. *Science Daily*, May 7. https://www.sciencedaily.com/releases/2015/02/1502 05123024.htm.

Leite, N. C., G. F. Salles, A. L. Araujo, C. A. Villela-Nogueira, and C. R. Cardoso. 2009. "Prevalence and Associated Factors of Non-alcoholic Fatty Liver Disease in Patients with Type-2 Diabetes Mellitus." *Liver International* 29 (1) (January): 113-19.

Ley, R. E., P. J. Turnbaugh, S. Klein, and J. L. Gordon. 2006. "Microbial Ecology: Human Gut Microbes Associated with Obesity." *Nature* 444 (7122) (December 21): 1022-23.

Li, J., N. Zhang, L. Hu, Z. Li, R. Li, C. Li, and S. Wang. 2011. "Improvement in Chewing Activity Reduces Energy Intake in One Meal and Modulates Plasma Gut Hormone Concentrations In Obese and Lean Young Chinese Men." *American Journal of Clinical Nutrition* 94 (3) (September): 709-16.

Liu, C. T., R. Raghu, S. H. Lin, S. Y. Wang, C. H. Kuo, Y. J. Tseng, and L. Y. Sheen. 2013. "Metabolomics of Ginger Essential Oil Against Alcoholic Fatty Liver in Mice." *Journal of Agricultural and Food Chemistry* 61 (46) (November 20): 11231-40.

Liu, W., S. S. Baker, R. D. Baker, and L. Zhu. 2015. "Antioxidant Mechanisms in Nonalcoholic Fatty Liver Disease." *Current Drug Targets* 16 (12): 1301-14.

Loguercio, C., A. Federico, C. Tuccillo, F. Terracciano, M. V. D'Auria, C. De Simone, and C. Del Vecchio Blanco. 2005. "Beneficial Effects of a Probiotic VSL#3 on Parameters of Liver Dysfunction in Chronic Liver Diseases." *Journal of Clinical Gastroenterology* 39 (6) (July): 540-43.

Loomba, R., C. B. Sirlin, J. B. Schwinner, and J. E. Lavine. 2009. "Advances in Pediatric Nonalcoholic Fatty Liver Disease." *Hepatology* 50 (4) (October): 1282-93.

Lustig, R. H., L. A. Schmidt, and C. D. Brindis. 2012. "Public Health: The Toxic Truth About Sugar." *Nature* 482 (February 2): 27-29.

Ma, J., C. S. Fox, P. F. Jacques, E. K. Speliotes, U. Hoffmann, C. E., Smith, E. Saltzman, and N. M. McKeown. 2015. "Sugar-Sweetened Beverage, Diet Soda, and Fatty Liver Disease in the Framingham Heart Study Cohorts." *Journal of Hepatology* 63 (2) (August): 462-69.

Ma, Y. Y., L. Li, C. H. Yu, Z. Shen, L. H. Chen, and Y. M. Li. 2013. "Effects of Probiotics on Nonalcoholic Fatty Liver Disease: A Meta-analysis." *World Journal of Gastroenterology* 19 (40) (October 28): 6911-18.

Malaguarnera, G., E. Cataudella, M. Giordano, G. Nunnari, G. Chisari, and M. Malaguarnera. 2012. "Toxic Hepatitis in Occupational Exposure to Solvents." *World Journal of Gastroenterology* 18 (22) (June 14): 2756-66.

Malaguarnera, M., M. Vacante, T. Antic, M. Giordano, G. Chisari, R. Acquaviva, S. Mastrojeni, G. Malaguarnera, A. Mistretta, G. Li Volti, and F. Galvano. 2012. "Bifidobacterium longum with Fructo-oligosaccharides in Patients with Non Alcoholic Steatohepatitis." *Digestive Diseases and Sciences* 57 (2) (February): 545-53.

Mandayam, S., M. M. Jamal, and T. R. Morgan. 2004. "Epidemiology of Alcoholic Liver Disease." *Seminars in Liver Disease* 24 (3) (August): 217-32.

Marikar, S., and L. Ferran. 2008. "Exclusive: Jeremy Piven Defends Play Departure Due to Mercury Poisoning." *ABC News*, January 15, 2008. http://abcnews.go.com/GMA/story?id=6652551.

Masterton, G. S., J. N. Plevris, and P. C. Hayes. 2010. "Review Article: Omega-3 Fatty Acids—A Promising Novel Therapy for Non-alcoholic Fatty Liver Disease." *Alimentary Pharmacology & Therapeutics* 31 (7): 679-692.

Mathurin, P., A. Hollebecque, L. Arnalsteen, D. Buob, E. Leteurtre, R. Caiazzo, M. Pigeyre, H. Verkindt, S. Dharancy, A. Louvet, M. Romon, and F. Pattou. 2009. "Prospective Study of the Long-Term Effects of Bariatric Surgery On Liver Injury in Patients Without Advanced Disease." *Gastroenterology* 137 (2) (August): 532-40.

Midanik, L. T. 1988. "Validity of Self-Reported Alcohol Use: A Literature Review and Assessment." *British Journal of Addiction* 83 (9) (September): 1019-30.

Miyake, T., T. Kumagi, M. Hirooka, S. Furukawa, K. Kawasaki, M. Koizumi, Y. Todo, S. Yamamoto, H. Nunoi, Y. Tokumoto, Y. Ikeda, M. Abe, K. Kitai, B. Matsuura, and Y. Hiasa. 2015. "Significance of Exercise in Nonalcoholic Fatty Liver Disease in Men: A Community-Based Large Cross-sectional Study." *Journal of Gastroenterology* 50 (2) (February): 230-37.

Mozaffarian, D., T. Hao, E. R. Rimm, W. C. Willett, and F. B. Hu. 2012. "Changes in Diet and Lifestyle and Long-Term Weight Gain in Women and Men." *New England Journal of Medicine* 364:2392-2404.

Mudipalli, A. "Lead Hepatoxicity & Potential Health Effects." 2007. *Indian Journal of Medical Research* 126 (6) (December): 518-27.

Muraki, E., Y. Hayashi, H. Chiba, N. Tsunoda, and K. Kasono. 2011. "Dose-Dependent Effects, Safety and Tolerability of Fenugreek in Diet-Induced Metabolic Disorders in Rats." *Lipids in Health and Disease* 10:240. http://www.ncbi.nlm.nih.gov/pmc/articles/PMC3292492/.

Murase, T., A. Nagasawa, J. Suzuki, T. Hase, and I. Tokimitsu. 2002. "Beneficial Effects of Tea Catechins on Diet-Induced Obesity: Stimulation of Lipid Catabolism in the Liver." *International Journal of Obesity* 26 (11) (November): 1459-64.

Musso, G., R. Gambino, M. Cassader, and G. Pagano. 2010. "A Meta-analysis of Randomized Trials for the Treatment of Nonalcoholic Fatty Liver Disease." *Hepatology* 52:79-104.

Nabavi, S. F., M. Daglia, A. H. Moghaddam, S. Habtemariam, and S. M. Nabavi. 2014. "Curcumin and Liver Disease: from Chemistry to Medicine." *Comprehensive Reviews in Food Science and Food Safety* 13 (1) (January): 62-77.

National Institute of Diabetes and Digestive and Kidney Diseases. LiverTox: Clinical and Research Information on Drug-Induced Liver Injury. http:// livertox.nlm.nih.gov/.

Nishioji, K., N. Mochizuki, M. Kobayashi, M. Kamaguchi, Y. Sumida, T. Nishimura, K. Yamaguchi, H. Kadotani, and Y. Itoh. 2015. "The Impact of PNPLA3 rs738409 Genetic Polymorphism and Weight Gain 10 kg After Age 20 on Non-Alcoholic Fatty Liver Disease in Non-Obese Japanese Individuals." *PLoS One* 20 (10) (October 20): e0140427.

"Nonalcoholic Fatty Liver: The New Face of Metabolic Syndrome." 2015. *Mayo Clinic Health Letter* 33 (2) (February): 1-3.

Noone, T. C., R. C. Semelka, D. M. Chaney, and C. Reinhold. 2004. "Abdominal Imaging Studies: Comparison of Diagnostic Accuracies Resulting from Ultrasound, Computed Tomography, and Magnetic Resonance Imaging in the Same Individual." *Magnetic Resonance Imaging* 22 (1) (January): 19-24.

Oh, S., T. Shida, K. Yamagishi, K. Tanaka, R. So, T. Tsujimoto, and J. Shoda. 2015. "Moderate to Vigorous Physical Activity Volume Is an Important Factor for Managing Nonalcoholic Fatty Liver Disease: A Retrospective Study." *Hepatology* 61 (4) (April): 1205-15.

Oh, S., K. Tanaka, E. Warabi, and J. Shoda. 2013. "Exercise Reduces Inflammation and Oxidative Stress in Obesity-Related Liver Diseases." *Medicine and Science in Sports and Exercise* 45 (12) (December): 2214-22.

Okla, M., I. Kang, D. M. Kim, V. Gourineni, N. Shay, L. Gu, and S. Chung. 2015. "Ellagic Acid Modulates Lipid Accumulation in Primary Human Adipocytes and Human Hepatoma Huh7 cells via Discrete Mechanisms." *Journal of Nutritional Biochemistry* 26 (1) (January): 82-90.

Oldways Preservation & Exchange Trust. Learn more about Oldways and the Mediterranean diet at www.oldwayspt.org

Ouyang, X., P. Cirillo, Y. Sautin, S. McCall, J. L. Bruchette, A. M. Diehl, R. J. Johnson, and M. J. Abdelmalek. 2008. "Fructose Consumption as a Risk Factor for Non-alcoholic Fatty Liver Disease." *Journal of Hepatology* 48 (6) (June): 993-99.

Paolella, G., C. Mandato, L. Pierri, M. Poeta, M. DiStasi, and P. Vajro. 2014. "Gut-Liver Axis and Probiotics: Their Role in Non-alcoholic Fatty Liver Disease." *World Journal of Gastroenterology* 20 (42) (November 14): 15518-31.

Parker, H. M., N. A. Johnson, C. A. Burdon, J. S. Cohn, H. T. O'Connor, and J. George. 2012. "Omega-3 Supplementation and Non-alcoholic Fatty Liver Disease: A Systematic Review and Meta-analysis." *Journal of Hepatology* 56 (4) (April): 944-951.

Pepino, M. Y., C. D. Tiemann, B. W. Patterson, B. M. Wice, and S. Klein. 2013. "Sucralose Affects Glycemic and Hormonal Responses to an Oral Glucose Load." *Diabetes Care* 36 (9) (April): 2530-35.

Piguet, A. C., U. Saran, C. Simillion, I. Keller, L. Terracciano, H. L. Reeves, and J. F. Dufour. 2015. "Regular Exercise Decreases Liver Tumors Development in Hepatocyte-Specific PTEN-Deficient Mice Independently of Steatosis." *Journal of Hepatology* 62 (6) (June): 1296-1303.

Pinto C. G., M. Marega, J. A. Carvalho, F. G. Carmona, C. E. Lopes, F. L. Ceschini, D. S. Bocalini, and A. J. Figueira Jr. 2015. "Physical Activity as a Protective Factor for Development of Non-alcoholic Fatty Liver in Men." *Einstein* 13 (1) (January-March): 34-40.

Polyzos, S. A., J. Kountouras, and M. A. Tsoukas. 2015. "Circulating Homocysteine in Nonalcoholic Fatty Liver Disease." *European Journal of Internal Medicine* 26 (2) March 1): 152-53.

Privitera, G. J., and H. E. Creary. 2012. "Proximity and Visibility of Fruits and Vegetables Influence Intake in a Kitchen Setting Among College Students." *Environment and Behavior* (April 17). Published online before print. http://eab.sagepub.com/content/45/7/876.

Purcell, K., P. Sumithran, L. A. Prendergast, C. J. Bouniu, E. Delbridge, and J. Proietto. 2014. "The Effect of Rate of Weight Loss on Long-Term Weight Management: A Randomized Controlled Trial." *Lancet: Diabetes & Endocrinology.* Published online (October 15). http://dx.doi.org/10.1016/S2213-8587(14)70200-1.

Rocha, R., H. P. Cotrim, A. C. Siqueira, and S. Floriano. 2007. "Non Alcoholic Fatty Liver Disease: Treatment with Soluble Fibres." *Arquivos de Gastroenterologia* 44 (4) (October-December): 350-52.

Rodríguez-Roisin, R., and M. J. Krowka. 2008. "Hepatopulmonary Syndrome—A Liver-Induced Lung Vascular Disorder." *New England Journal of Medicine* 358 (May 29): 2378-87.

Rogers, M. A., and D. M. Aronoff. 2016. "The Influence of Non-steroidal Anti-Inflammatory Drugs on the Gut Microbiome." *Clinical Microbiology and Infection* 22 (2) (February): 178.

Russ, T. C., M. Kivimäki, J. R. Morling, J. M. Starr, E. Stamatakis, and G. D. Batty. 2015. "Association Between Psychological Distress and Liver Disease Mortality: A Meta-analysis of Individual Study Participants." *Gastroenterology* 148:958-66.

Sabry, A. A., M. A. Sobh, W. L. Irving, A. Grabowska, B. E. Wagner, S. Fox, G. Kudesia, and A. M. El Nahas. 2002. "A Comprehensive Study of the Association Between Hepatitis C Virus and Glomerulopathy." *Nephrology Dialysis Transplantation* 17 (2): 239-45.

Saich, R., and R. Chapman. 2008 "Primary Sclerosing Cholangitis, Autoimmune

Hepatitis and Overlap Syndromes in Inflammatory Bowel Disease." *World Journal of Gastroenterology* 14 (3) (January 21): 331-37.

Sanyal, A. J., N. Chalasani, K. V. Kowdley, A. McCullough, A. M. Diehl, N. M. Bass, B. A. Neuschwander-Tetri, J. E. Lavine, J. Tonascia, A. Unalp, M. Van Natta, J. Clark, E. M. Brunt, D. E. Kleiner, J. H. Hoofnagle, and P. R. Robuck. 2010. "Pioglitazone, Vitamin E, or Placebo for Nonalcoholic Steatohepatitis." *New England Journal of Medicine* 362 (May 6): 1675-85

Schiff, E. R., W. C. Maddrey, and M. F. Sorrell. 2011. *Schiff's Diseases of the Liver*, 11th ed. Hoboken, NJ: Wiley-Blackwell.

Schwimmer, J. B., C. Behling, R. Newbury, R. Deutsch, C. Nievergelt, N. J. Schork, and J. E. Lavine. 2005. "Histopathology of Pediatric Nonalcoholic Fatty Liver Disease." *Hepatology* 42 (3) (September): 641-49.

Schwimmer, J. B., R. Deutsch, T. Kahen, J. E. Lavine, C. Stanley, C. Behling. 2006. "Prevalence of Fatty Liver in Children and Adolescents." *Pediatrics* 118 (4) (October): 1388-93.

Schwimmer, J. B., N. McGreal, R. Deutsch, M. J. Finegold, and J. E. Lavine.2005. "Influence of Gender, Race, and Ethnicity on Suspected Fatty Liver in Obese Adolescents." *Pediatrics* 115 (5) (May): e561-e565.

Schwimmer, J. B., M. S. Middleton, C. Behling, K. P. Newton, H. I. Awai, M. N. Paiz, J. Lam, J. C. Hooker, G. Hamilton, J. Fontanesi, and C. B. Sirlin. 2015. "Magnetic Resonance Imaging and Liver Histology as Biomarkers of Hepatic Steatosis in Children with Nonalcoholic Fatty Liver Disease." *Hepatology* 61 (6) (June): 1887-95.

Shamsoddini, A., V. Sobhani, M. E. Chamar Chehreh, S. M. Alavian, and A. Zaree. 2015. "Effect of Aerobic and Resistance Exercise Training on Liver Enzymes and Hepatic Fat in Iranian Men with Nonalcoholic Fatty Liver Disease." *Hepatitis Monthly* 15 (10) (October 10): e31434.

Shapiro, A., W. Mu, C. Roncal, K.-Y. Cheng, R. J. Johnson, and P. J. Scarpace. 2008. "Fructose-Induced Leptin Resistance Exacerbates Weight Gain in Response to Subsequent High-Fat Feeding." *American Journal of Physiology: Regulatory, Integrative and Comparative Physiology* 295 (5) (November 1): R1370-R1375.

Sharifi, N., R. Amani, E. Jahiani, and B. Cheraghian. 2014. "Does Vitamin D Improve Liver Enzymes, Oxidative Stress, and Inflammatory Biomarkers in Adults with Non-alcoholic Fatty Liver Disease? A Randomized Clinical Trial." *Endocrine* 47 (1) (September): 70-80.

Sharma, K. K., U. K. T. Prasada, and P. Kumar. 2014. "A Study on the Effect of Yoga Therapy on Liver Functions." *European Scientific Journal* 10 (6) (February): 246-51.

Sharma, V., G. Shashank, and S. Aggarwal. 2013. "Probiotics and Liver Disease." *Permanente Journal* 17 (4) (Fall): 62-67.

Shimazu, T., Y. Tsubono, S. Kuriyama, K. Ohmori, Y. Koizumi, Y. Nishino, D. Shibuya, and I. Tsuji. 2005. "Coffee Consumption and the Risk of Primary Liver Cancer: Pooled Analysis of Two Prospective Studies in Japan." *International Journal of Cancer* 116 (1) (August 10): 150–54.

Slack, A., A. Yeoman, and J. Wendon. 2010. "Renal Dysfunction in Chronic Liver Disease." *Critical Care* 14 (2) (March 9): 214.

Sreenivasa Baba, C., G. Alexander, B. Kalyani, R. Pandey, S. Rastogi, A. Pandey, and G. Choudhuri. 2006. "Effect of Exercise and Dietary Modification on Serum Aminotransferase Levels in Patients with Nonalcoholic Steatohepatitis." *Journal of Gastroenterology and Hepatology* 21 (1 Pt 1) (January): 191–98.

Targher, G., C. P. Day, and E. Bonora. 2010. "Risk of Cardiovascular Disease in Patients with Nonalcoholic Fatty Liver Disease." *New England Journal of Medicine* 363 (September 30): 1341–50.

Tremaroli, V., and F. Bäckhed. 2012. "Functional Interactions Between the Gut Microbiota and Host Metabolism." *Nature* 489 (7415) (September 13): 242–49.

Trovato, F. M., D. Catalano, G. F. Martines, P. Pace, and G. M. Trovato. 2015. "Mediterranean Diet and Non-alcoholic Fatty Liver Disease: The Need of Extended and Comprehensive Interventions." *Clinical Nutrition* 34 (1) (February): 86–88.

Valenti, L., P. Riso, A. Mazzocchi, M. Porrini, S. Fargion, and C. Agostoni, C. 2013. "Dietary Anthocyanins as Nutritional Therapy for Nonalcoholic Fatty Liver Disease." *Oxidative Medicine and Cellular Longevity* 2013: 145421.

Valtueña, S., N. Pellegrini, D. Ardigò, D. Del Rio, F. Numeroso, F. Scazzina, L. Monti, I. Zavaroni, and F. Brighenti. 2006. "Dietary Glycemic Index and Liver Steatosis." *American Journal of Clinical Nutrition* 84 (1) (July): 136–42.

Vos, M. B., and J. E. Lavine. 2013. "Dietary Fructose in Nonalcoholic Fatty Liver Disease." *Hepatology* 57 (6) (June): 2525–31.

Wahlang, B., J. I. Beier, H. B. Clair, H. J. Bellis-Jones, K. C. Falkner, C. J. McClain, and M. C. Cave. 2013. "Toxicant-Associated Steatohepatitis." *Toxicologic Pathology* 41 (2) (February): 343–60.

Wang, R., R. Koretz, and H. Yee. 2003. "Is Weight Reduction an Effective Therapy for Nonalcoholic Fatty Liver? A Systematic Review." *American Journal of Medicine* 115:554–59.

Wansink, B. 2007. *Mindless Eating: Why We Eat More Than We Think.* New York: Bantam.

Wansink, B. 2014. *Slim By Design: Mindless Eating Solutions for Everyday Life.* New York: William Morrow.

Wigg, A. J., I. C. Roberts-Thomson, R. B. Dymock, P. J. McCarthy, R. H. Grose, and A. G. Cummins. 2001. "The Role of Small Intestinal Bacterial Overgrowth, Intestinal Permeability, Endotoxaemia, and Tumour Necrosis Factor α in the Pathogenesis of Non-alcoholic Steatohepatitis." *Gut* 48 (2) (February): 206-11.

Willis, B. L., A. Gao, D. Leonard, L. F. DeFina, and J. D. Berry. 2012. "Midlife Fitness and the Development of Chronic Conditions in Later Life." *Archives of Internal Medicine* 172 (17) (September 24): 1333-40.

Xia, W., Y. Jiang, Y. Li, Y. Wan, J. Liu, Y. Ma, Z. Mao, H. Chang, G. Li, B. Xu, X. Chen, and S. Xu. 2014. "Early-Life Exposure to Bisphenol A Induces Liver Injury in Rats Involvement of Mitochondria-Mediated Apoptosis." *PLoS One* 9 (2): e90443.

Xiao, Q., R. Sinha, B. I. Graubard, and N. D. Freedman. 2014. "Inverse Associations of Total and Decaffeinated Coffee With Liver Enzyme Levels in National Health and Nutrition Examination Survey 1999-2010." *Hepatology* 60 (6) (December): 2091-98.

Yang, Q. 2010. "Gain Weight by 'Going Diet?' Artificial Sweeteners and the Neurobiology of Sugar Cravings." *Yale Journal of Biology and Medicine* 83 (2) (June): 101-8.

Yoga Journal. "Poses for Your Liver." http://www.yogajournal.com/category/poses/anatomy/liver/.

Yu, D., X.-O. Shu, Y.-B. Xiang, H. Li, G. Yang, Y.-T. Gao, W. Zheng, and X. Zhang. 2014. "Higher Dietary Choline Intake Is Associated with Lower Risk of Nonalcoholic Fatty Liver in Normal-Weight Chinese Women." *The Journal of Nutrition* 144 (12) (December 1): 2034-40.

Yuan, H., J. Y.-J. Shyy, and M. Martins-Green. 2009. "Second-Hand Smoke Stimulates Lipid Accumulation in the Liver by Modulating AMPK and SREBP-1." *Journal of Hepatology* 51 (3) (September): 535-47.

Zelber-Sagi, S., A. Buch, H. Yeshua, N. Vaisman, M. Webb, G. Harari, O. Kis, N. Fliss-Isakov, E. Izhakov, A. Halpern, E. Santo, R. Oren, and O. Shibolet. 2014. "Effect of Resistance Training on Non-alcoholic Fatty-Liver Disease: A Randomized-Clinical Trial." *World Journal of Gastroenterology* 20 (15) (April 21): 4382-92.

Zelber-Sagi, S., D. Nitzan-Kaluski, R. Goldsmith, M. Webb, I. Zvibel, I. Goldiner, L. Blendis, Z. Halpern, and R. Oren, R. 2008. "Role of Leisure-Time Physical Activity in Nonalcoholic Fatty Liver Disease: A Population-Based Study." *Hepatology* 48 (6) (December): 1791-98.

Zheng, Z., X. Zhang, J. Wang, A. Dandekar, H. Kim, Y. Qiu, X. Xu, Y. Cui, A. Wang, L. C. Chen, S. Rajagopalan, Q. Sun, and K. Zhang. 2015. "Exposure to Fine Airborne Particulate Matters Induces Hepatic Fibrosis in Murine Models." *Journal of Hepatology* 63 (6) (December): 1397-1404.

Zimmerman, A. 2004. "Regulation of Liver Regeneration." *Nephrology Dialysis Transplantation* 19 (Suppl. 4): iv6-iv10.

recipe index

index